Opening
the
Gate of Life

Wisdom for Cultivating
Health, Vitality, and Longevity

David Goodell, M.Ac.

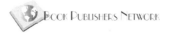 BOOK PUBLISHERS NETWORK

Book Publishers Network
P.O. Box 2256
Bothell • WA • 98041
Ph • 425-483-3040
www.bookpublishersnetwork.com

10 9 8 7 6 5 4 3 2 1

Printed in the United States of America

LCCN 2013934578
ISBN 978-1-937454-76-0

Photo of David Goodell by Poppy Barach.
Interior design by Stephanie Martindale.
Cover design by Laura Zugzda.
Photos of Cheng Man-Ch"ing by Kenneth Van Sickle.
Photo of J. R. Worsley by Steven Flores.
Photo of Patrick Watson by Pat Gorman.
Photo of Oscar Ichazo courtesy of Arica Institute.
Layers of Chi and Bites Out of Our Chi illustrations adapted with permission from originals by Pat Gorman.
All other photos, charts, and illustrations by David Goodell.

Publisher's Cataloging-in-Publication
(Provided by Quality Books, Inc.)

Goodell, David.
Opening the Gate of Life: Wisdom for cultivating health,
vitality and longevity. / by David Goodell.
p. cm.
Includes bibliographical references.
ISBN 978-1-937454-76-0
1. Health. I. Title.
RA776.G66 2011   613
QBI11-600112

For Michael and Esther

Contents

Foreword

This book is meant for those who know, or are beginning to suspect, that living in harmony with ourselves, our neighbors, other life on the planet, and of course, with the earth are more than ideals. They are essential prerequisites to our health and humanity's survival.

Furthermore, it is increasingly clear that while those of us in the healing professions can help alleviate suffering, there is little that we can actually cure. Nature within and around us is the healer, and an unbelievably powerful one at that. Our job as patients and as health-care providers is to assist nature in doing its work. The first step is a practical and realistic understanding of how nature works.

The knowledge offered in this book is rooted in ancient traditions, increasingly validated by current scientific research. It is indispensable for becoming and staying well and for helping others do the same.

Anecdotes are given to illustrate some of the points along with practical and enjoyable ways of employing this wisdom. A bibliography at the end provides further sources of information.

Introduction

I have been treating patients as an acupuncturist since 1985, twenty-eight years now. Over that time, I have treated people with many different illnesses, including AIDS, allergies of every sort, anxiety, arthritis, asthma, attention deficit disorder, auto immune disorders, cancer, chronic fatigue, chronic infections, clinical depression, Crohn's disease, diabetes, drug addiction, eating disorders, hypertension, insomnia, pain of all kinds, and injuries, both emotional and physical, that couldn't seem to heal. The list goes on from there.

I have been astonished at how resilient we are when we understand and work with the natural laws governing our body, mind, and spirit. Time and again, I have seen people heal from such severe illness and injury that I would not have thought becoming well again was possible. Our natural, innate resilience gives me tremendous hope, especially for those patients who are very ill.

I am also alarmed at how divorced from reality our cultural assumptions about health have become. We have temporarily achieved a high material standard of living, but our lack of understanding about our essential nature and how we are an integral part of the oneness of the creation has made us among the sickest and least happy people in the world. We are destroying the environment, our sources of clean food and water, and many other species in our quest for amusement, security, material wealth, and comfort. In the process, we are also destroying ourselves.

We spend almost twice as much per capita on health care as any other country, yet the incidence of cancer, heart disease, diabetes, drug abuse, depression, and so on continues to rise. Lacking a real understanding and means for actually becoming well again, more of us are taking more medications than ever before and expect to take them for life. The long-term side effects are damaging to our health. Medication residues in our urine become pollutants in our water. And, we continue to become more ill at ease, sicker, and unhappier.

Rather than resign yourself to this path, I encourage you to consider a broader view of health and well-being than is propagated by mass media and advertising paid for by the drug industry. There are times when the strong interventions western medicine can provide are beneficial and lifesaving. Thank God for them. However, regaining and maintaining our best possible health requires living in balance with the natural laws that govern how our bodies work in harmony with the world and the people around us. Living in balance requires a clear-eyed understanding of these natural laws.

This book offers practical information about health, vitality, and quality of life. Rooted in sophisticated traditions, it is a concise summary of the fundamentals of cultivating your vitality and opening the gate of life. With a little understanding and enjoyable effort, we can reap a rich harvest of feeling our best, regaining our health when possible, and feeling more at ease than we ever have, regardless of our age or stage in life.

I encourage you to take heart and help yourself become and stay well.

May the wisdom you gain
benefit you and every living being.

Chapter 1

Awakening

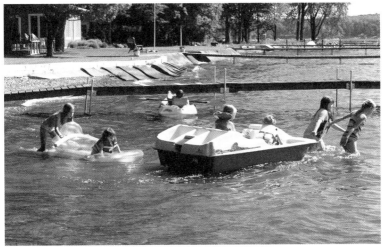

Children playing in Chautauqua Lake, New York.

My four brothers and I grew up in a small house next to Chautauqua Lake in a beautiful, semi-rural area of western New York. We enjoyed a large extended family of wonderful, kind, successful people who were actively involved in the community. Our home was a haven for kids. Cousins and friends often stayed with us for extended periods over the summers. We spent countless hours outside all year round.

By age ten, I was reading about Native Americans and how conscious they were of the weather, the seasons, the earth, and the plants, animals, and people around them. They understood and respected nature. Seeing the lake become increasingly polluted, I realized that we were largely ignoring the balance of nature.

By 1971, at age nineteen, I was questioning the cultural beliefs and values that shape the way we live. We were embroiled in the Vietnam War, and although I initially thought stopping the spread of communism justified the war, I was having doubts. About that time, two close friends, Tom Hetzel and Gary Hallberg, moved from our sleepy little town to the Big Apple to begin their meditation studies with the Arica Institute, a School of Knowledge founded in 1968 by philosopher Oscar Ichazo. When they told me about it, I thought they must have taken LSD and gone round the bend.

Personal setbacks over the next two years brought me to a deep state of disillusionment. I could see that, while several of the musicians I had been playing with had found their path in life, music was not going to be mine. My parents were getting a divorce. I had lost interest in my major in college. I had concluded that the Vietnam War was a terrible blunder, and I was about to get drafted. My lottery number was fifty. Had the war continued I would have been drafted within a couple of months. The last straw was losing the young woman with whom I was living to another man. I stopped sleeping. I had no interest in food or anything else. I was thoroughly demoralized and discouraged. I felt I did not fit anywhere.

After about three weeks of this, I realized that, while I was intensely unhappy about how things were going, those things were not the cause of my suffering. I was suffering because of my thoughts and feelings about what was happening. I felt these events were somehow wrong; they should not be happening. This feeling was the product of my unexamined beliefs, assumptions, and limited understanding of life.

This led me to speak with my friends Tom and Gary, who had gone through similar disillusionment before beginning their meditation work with Arica. They invited me to New York City, where two weeks later I attended my first Arica training. My perspective and the course of my life changed. I deeply appreciate them and the Arica school for that.

I began my studies with Arica Institute in 1973. By 1975, I had moved to Arlington, Virginia, to continue the Arica work with a community of like-minded people there. Later that year, about forty of us began to study T'ai Chi with the newly formed School of T'ai Chi Chuan, founded by Patrick Watson, a student in the Arica School and a senior student with Professor Cheng Man-ch'ing.

While continuing my studies with Arica and the School of T'ai Chi Chuan, I was introduced to Classical Five Element Acupuncture teachings of J. R. Worsley. I studied extensively with J. R. Worsley from 1984 until his death in 2003, and with Judy Becker Worsley, his successor, until 2008.

The roots of these traditions go back to the Yellow Emperor (ca 2500 BC) of China, whose discovery of the unity of the creation provided the foundation of Taoism, Confucianism, T'ai Chi, and Classical Five Element Acupuncture. These are the jewels of Chinese culture and the cohesive force that was the foundation of a civilization remarkable for periods of stability, harmony, peace, and prosperity lasting thousands of years.[1]

Oscar Ichazo's work, presented through the Arica Institute, builds on the work of the Taoists, the great Greek and Buddhist philosophers, and modern western knowledge of anatomy, physiology, and psychology to provide a complete map of the human psyche and a precise new method of achieving enlightenment that is original to him.

Most of the information in this book comes from these traditions and my experience studying, practicing, meditating, treating patients, and teaching over these past thirty-seven years.

I have witnessed the wisdom from these traditions help many people become more alive, aware of the preciousness of life, healthier, and happier. Through using these principles and practices daily, I am able to function much more efficiently and enjoy much better vitality. In short, they give me back many times what I put in.

I hope this book helps you awaken to the possibility of trusting and working wisely with nature within and around you to feel your best.

Chapter Notes

[1] Over the past five thousand years, the understanding of the oneness, or unity of the creation, realized by the Yellow Emperor has been further articulated and applied to everyday life by the great sages of ancient China.

Chi Po, the Yellow Emperor's physician, is thought to have written the *Yellow Emperor's Classic on Internal Medicine.* This text provides the foundation for Classical Five Element Acupuncture. Fu Xi is believed to have written the *I Ching,* known in the West as the *Book of Changes,* around 2000 BC. Rather than the basis of the parlor game of throwing pennies to foretell one's future, as it is commonly misunderstood, the *I Ching* describes all of the possible situations or phases of change and what will inevitably follow.

Around 770 BC, towards the end of the Zhou Dynasty, its emperor was said to have lost his virtue and, with it, the Mandate of Heaven to rule. China became fragmented, with various states vying for power, and descended into a period of civil war known as the Warring States period (471–221 BC).

Seeing the loss of harmony with the unity of the creation and seeking to re-establish its principles, the legendary Taoist sage Lao Tzu is said to have written the *Tao Te Ching* around 500 BC. Confucius was born in 551 BC during the turmoil leading to the Warring States period. His mission was to help restore social harmony by teaching about ethical human relationships. He and his students are thought to have authored *The Doctrine of the Mean, The Great Learning*, and *The Analects.* Sun Tzu, a general, wrote *The Art of War* around 500 BC. This text applies Taoist principles to restore harmony and bring conflict to its least destructive conclusion. Because the principles Sun Tzu taught are timeless, *The Art of War* is still studied as a military classic.

Qin Shi Huang, ruler of the largest state, conquered the rival states in 221 BC and established the Qin Dynasty. To unite the empire and end dissent, he ordered most of the books of the ancient sages burned and those who spoke of their contents executed. During the eleven years he reigned, many ancient texts were lost. Those who understood the wisdom of the early sages and lived to teach about it later passed it on after Qin Shi Huang's rule ended. This is one of the reasons why the history of the early sages and their writings are the subject of so much debate by modern scholars.

My belief, supported by my experience, is that the essence of these teachings has indeed been preserved and deepened. This wisdom has been made available through the master teachers (and others) from whom I have had the great good fortune of learning what is outlined in this book.

Chapter 2

The Tao

Life-giving processes are neither static nor linear, but cyclical and always in motion. We breathe in; then we breathe out. The sun rises, progresses across the sky, then sets. The seasons follow an orderly progression as well. Seeing every process as cyclical is necessary if we are to understand reality as it actually is, continuously in motion.

Furthermore, the points of change between one state of being and another are not random, but orderly and inherent in every aspect of the creation. Seeing and understanding the cyclical movement between already established points of change makes it possible to function accurately and efficiently in the world.

We are inseparable from nature. The cycles that occur in nature not only affect us; they also occur within us. Understanding these cycles and the points of change within them is fundamental to living a balanced, healthy life.

The sages of ancient China had a profoundly clear and accurate way of describing this. They saw the creation as one thing, arising from a timeless, inexhaustible source that cannot be named.

They saw the cyclical movement within the creation as everything alternates between apparent opposites—dark and light, cold and hot, matter and energy, female and male—and called these apparent opposites yin and yang.

The yin/yang symbol pictured below illustrates this understanding. Progressing clockwise around the circle shows the movement within the Oneness as yin (shown in black) gives way to yang (shown in white) and vice versa.

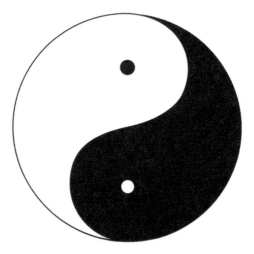

Yin/Yang Symbol

When yang reaches the peak of predominance, it invariably starts to give way to yin. Similarly, yin will eventually manifest fully again as the unbroken flow between yin and yang continues. The ocean water level rises until high tide and then begins to recede. Once low tide is reached, the tide starts coming in again.

Furthermore, everything contains the seed of its apparent opposite. This is represented by the black dot in the midst of the most yang portion, symbolizing the seed of yin, yang's apparent opposite, and by the white dot in the center of the black portion. There is shade during the day; the moon and stars provide a bit of light at night. There are a few sunny, relatively warm days in winter; summer has its cool rainy days too. Waves momentarily raise the water level at low tide and lower it during high tide.

The Five Elements

The ancients recognized that everything—all of the material stuff we see as well as every living being—is a manifestation of the One. All come into their current form and eventually dissolve into formlessness through the endless cycle of yin and yang moving through five distinct phases. The ancients called these five phases the five elements. The movement of yin and yang through the five elements, or phases of yin and yang, is shown below.

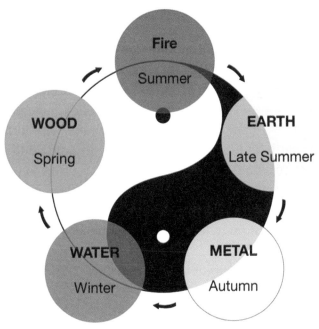

The Five Elements

These five phases, or five elements, are perhaps most easily seen in the five seasons: winter, spring, summer, late summer, and autumn.

Winter, the coldest, darkest, most yin time of year, corresponds to the water element. Rain and snow replenish the reservoirs. Nature seems to be at rest, gathering its strength.

Spring, gaining warmth and light, corresponds to the wood element, so called because of the burst of new growth in nature. Life is asserting itself again with all the energy, hopefulness, and vitality of a fresh start.

Summer, the most yang, corresponds to the fire element. The warmth, the light, and the long days provide the energy for the plants and animals to mature into adulthood.

Late summer corresponds to the earth element. The heat of summer is waning, and the earth is producing a harvest that will sustain us through the coming winter.

Autumn, as daylight further shortens, corresponds to the metal element. Nature lets go of what has served its purpose. The leaves and foliage drop to the ground, enriching the soil with trace minerals and organic matter.

This cycle can be seen in every process, including the stages of life. We sprout from a tiny seed, which lies dormant until fertilized. We grow with the amazing vitality of youth. We gain strength and knowledge as we mature into adulthood. We produce a body of work and sufficient harvest to provide for ourselves and perhaps a family, while setting something aside for our later years. At the conclusion of our life's work, we pass our best on to the next generation and let go of what is no longer needed.

Seeing these stages of life's cycle makes it easier to live in harmony with them. Recognizing that each is beautiful and appropriate at the proper time lessens the desire to be in a hurry to get to the next stage, attempt to remain in one stage after it has passed, or to dread what will come next.

Even death is as sacred and natural a part of life as birth. Pure spirit enters our body at birth and leaves at death. Understanding the stages of life helps us enjoy each of them and live a full and productive life.

The sages referred to the practice of living in harmony with the Oneness of the Creation and its cycles as following the Tao.

Chapter 3

Chi

The ancient Chinese sages understood that the whole creation is permeated with, held together with, and moved by energy.

Our life is possible because of the vital energy, or "chi," that circulates within us. It is the energy we need to move, think, grow, and feel. It enables our bodies to repair and maintain themselves and to heal from injury and illness, including emotional distress. It is our most valuable resource. Once we have used up our chi, our life comes to an end.

For thousands of years, Chinese culture has refined an understanding of chi. T'ai Chi Chuan (now commonly referred to as simply "T'ai Chi") and Qi Gong, the slow, gentle series of movements you may have seen Chinese people practicing together in parks, as well as Classical Five Element Acupuncture, are all rooted in a sophisticated understanding of the natural laws that govern the flow of chi within us and provide precise means of balancing and cultivating our chi.

Despite experiencing the profound benefits of T'ai Chi and Classical Five Element Acupuncture, I needed some time to understand and grasp the significance of this vital chi energy. My western understanding held no frame of reference for chi and its importance for my health.

I learned in school that the universe is composed of matter and energy and that moving matter requires an expenditure of energy. I could see that energy is necessary for moving about in the world but did not see the connection between our energy and our health.

From our western perspective, it is perfectly reasonable to attribute disease to physical things like germs, poor nutrition, toxins, injuries, or genetics. We attribute mental and emotional problems to chemical imbalances within our bodies as well. Therefore, we expect treatment by physical means: nutrition, chemicals, and surgery.

As I have matured, my narrow understanding of health as based on physical conditions has opened into a broader view. We now know that matter (even that which we take to be solid) is almost entirely space. Hydrogen, for example, is the most common element on earth, a component of water and nearly every organic compound. Its atoms each have an electron and a proton. If we were to take a hydrogen atom and expand it to the size of a football stadium, the "solid" portion, the proton, would be roughly the size of an orange in the center of the stadium. The electron would be about the size of a grape seed zipping around the proton somewhere inside the stadium. The rest is space. The electron doesn't fly away because it is held within this space by energy.

Explorations outside the earth's atmosphere, where there is almost no matter, have revealed that space is not actually empty. A vast amount of energy streams continuously through it in the form of light, heat, and electromagnetic radiation. The planets are held in their orbits by the gravitational pull, another form of energy, from the sun.

In short, the universe is filled with and held together by energy. Even what seems to be solid matter is almost entirely space permeated with energy. The idea of "solid" matter is only a construction of our mind.

Energy takes many forms. The energy in sunlight contains many wavelengths and can be separated by a prism into a rainbow of color. Other manifestations of energy have wavelengths that are above or below the visual spectrum. Energy can be stored in plants, for example, or coal, oil, or radioactive materials. Some of those forms are unsuitable or even toxic for our bodies. Enriched uranium can provide the energy that lights a city, but even a minute bit will kill us.

The energy, or chi, that gives us life is specific and must come in a form that meets our needs. We acquire our chi through our favorable interaction with the sun, earth, air, water, plants, and other forms of life around us.

Whereas the ancient sages recognized that we are inseparable from nature around us, our western culture has generally viewed the creation around us as something to be tamed, conquered, and bent to our will. The ancient sages understood that our chi comes from the world around us and that our health depends on living in harmony with the chi that permeates the creation, both inside and outside of us. They understood that all of nature, including us, is part of one fabric.

In contrast, we in the West tend to have the adversarial view of "us versus the natural world." Whereas the ancient sages looked to balancing our chi as the primary means of restoring our health, we see disease as something foreign that we need to fight. Our medicine helps us fight infection, fight cancer, fight depression, fight high blood pressure, fight diabetes, and in general, fight disease.

Using physical medicine to combat disease, based on the concept of disease as having material causes, functions effectively up to a point. Many lives have been saved with antibiotics, surgery, radiation, chemotherapy, and other medications. However, the fight also turns our bodies into a battleground and inflicts considerable collateral damage.

Successful medical treatment may help us overcome an illness and even save our life, but it rarely brings us to an optimum state of health where we are naturally vibrant, happy, and energetic again. Nor does it restore our natural immunity and resilience.

The idea that disease arises from material problems does not fully explain the causes of disease or how to restore a person to his or her optimum health. It has become clear to me that a realistic understanding of life and health also requires a deeper understanding of the vital chi energy that holds us together, connects us with the rest of the creation, and enables our body, mind, and spirit to function.

The universe behaves according to natural laws. For example, we know that water always boils at a particular temperature and pressure, materials have their tensile strength, and chemical reactions occur under specific, repeatable conditions. The laws of physics, chemistry, and thermodynamics are consistent and impersonal. All of our science and technology is based on understanding the natural laws that govern how the material world functions.

Natural laws also govern how our chi functions within us. Once we recognize that our bodies are mostly space, held together by the energy, or chi, inside us, we are ready to examine, as the ancient sages have, the natural laws that govern how we can nourish and balance our chi.

A clear understanding and practical means of taking care of the life-giving vital chi energy that we need to sustain us is indispensable for getting better if we are sick and then living a full and healthy life once we are well. I have come to see balancing and nourishing our chi as the most important means of taking care of ourselves.

Chapter 4
Age and Illness

Our understanding of health, aging, and illness is based upon many unexamined beliefs that we have come to accept without question. One is the assumption that our bodies function in a mechanical way. As Oscar Ichazo wrote in the introduction to his book, *Master Level Exercise: Psychocalisthenics*:

> [Health is the result of] an enormously complex process ... a delicate balance of several variables that works at once producing transformations triggered by hormones, enzymes, vitamins, minerals, and that indescribable energy known in ancient China as "chi", broadly translated as vital energy, and linked with the energy of our surroundings and ... with the entire universe.
>
> We [in the West] consider normal the standard collapse of [our bodies], struck by the symptoms of old age: hardening of the arteries, irregular blood pressure, ineptitude of the organism for metabolizing sugar, ineptitude for breaking down protein molecules, shrinking of the encephalon, losing sharpness of memory, imagination, senses

and will to live, and consequently poor digestion and absorption, constipation, arthritis, obesity, and collapsing of the muscular tone that ultimately affects the heart.

What is imperative for us to consider is how, by what means, can we stop this process of decay that we see as being part of our natural life as human beings. This we have to emphasize, because this type of decay, decrepitude and senility … is unknown in wildlife.

The gradual decline we in the west accept and attribute to aging is not seen in the animal kingdom, where the animals function at a consistently high level until shortly before their death. We can object that in nature, animals, when losing agility, will simply perish. This is true, but it seems that nature triggers old age at once. For example, the salmon, as we know, proves to be at the top of his vitality and strength when returning to the stream of his origin, where he will reproduce. Within a few hours, he will decay and with surprising speed die … and not in the form of a slow and endless agony, as we are accustomed to accept as part of the lifespan of human beings.

We accept old age as a fate from which nobody seems to be free.

Nobody? That does not seem to be the case in the lives of many individuals who have devoted their existence to perfecting themselves and their society. There is a similarity between their lives and the life of the salmon: it is in their last years that they become more productive and a positive

influence for their fellow human beings. As in the
case of the salmon, they suddenly stop producing,
have a fast decay, and die. Take, for example, the
lives of great artists, scientists, and mystics, many
… producing at the best of their ability until the
very end, when suddenly they collapse and die.
Richard Strauss described this situation as a soft
and kind desire to go to sleep—simple and natural.

I believe that we are old souls and that we have been through
the cycle of birth, childhood, young adult, mature adult, parent,
teacher, mentor, wise old age, and death many times.

Regardless of whether this is true, I find it a useful way
of seeing the various stages of life and what is appropriate for
each stage. As we age and mature, we are ready for increasing levels of responsibility. Some responsibilities, like being
a parent, require more physical stamina and are better suited
for a younger person. Others, like being a teacher, mentor, or
leader, require the knowledge, experience, and wisdom that
come from living longer.

Losing our vitality and clarity as we age results in a tremendous waste of the wisdom that older people can contribute to
their family, community, and society.

In my experience, a consistent, easy daily practice of cultivating our chi is the most potent means of becoming and
remaining well, capable of functioning at a high level well into
old age. It is the antidote to the gradual decline we so often see
as time goes by and mistakenly attribute to old age.

Chi and Health

Our well-being, as the ancient sages realized, is the result of
abundant chi flowing within us in a state of balance that sustains
our health. Our chi circulates within our bodies along pathways

called meridians, which connect every internal organ, tissue, and cell, providing the energy that makes every living function possible. It provides the energy our bodies need to repair and maintain themselves.

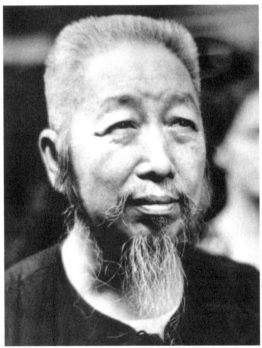

Professor Cheng Man-ch'ing. (Photo by Kenneth Van Sickle.)

The importance of a daily practice of replenishing and circulating our chi cannot be overemphasized. It is tempting to think, "This all sounds good in theory, but come on. How much of a difference can this really make?"

The late Professor Cheng was in his twenties when he contracted tuberculosis. At the time, in the 1920s, it was a death sentence. His teeth had become loose, and he was coughing up blood when he was accepted as a student of Yang Cheng Fu, a renowned T'ai Chi master. Professor Cheng practiced his

T'ai Chi from morning until night, when exhausted, he would collapse onto his bed.

Over the next several months, he overcame the disease. Once he became well, he discontinued his T'ai Chi practice. Within a few years, he again contracted tuberculosis. He again took up T'ai Chi and again regained his health. After this happened a third time, he resumed his T'ai Chi practice and never missed a day.

He later wrote, "Heaven sent me illness after illness to cure me of my indolence."

Professor Cheng went on to become a renowned master of Five Excellences—Chinese poetry, painting, calligraphy, medicine (he was the equivalent of the surgeon general of China under Chiang Kai Chiak), and T'ai Chi Chuan. He enjoyed good health, vigor, and productivity until he died in his seventies.

In looking at the process of illness, when our chi becomes blocked or exhausted, the first thing that generally happens is we don't feel so happy and energetic. Our bodies don't function as well as they should. Our appetite may go out of proportion, we may not sleep well, we may feel frustrated, anxious, or depressed, and our mental clarity suffers. If the imbalance continues, our bodies fall into disrepair. Eventually, we become sick and die.

So, we have two fundamental tasks if we wish to feel our best. First, we must keep the flow of energy within us balanced and moving freely. Second, we need to maintain an abundant supply of our chi because, while the energy of the creation is inexhaustible, the chi inside us is not.

Chapter 5
Chi Equation

The "Chi Equation" is a way of seeing how much chi we are taking in compared to how much chi we are using up. It helps us understand how to maintain an abundant supply of chi inside us.

We have three sources of chi:

    a. The air we breathe,
    b. The food we eat, and
    c. What we have inherited from our parents—our ancestral chi.

Everything we do requires some of our chi—growing, thinking, talking, working, and so on. When we use more chi than we are able to replenish by the food we eat and the air we breathe, we make up the difference by tapping into our ancestral chi. Once our ancestral chi is exhausted, our life comes to an end.

If we wish to live a full and healthy life, we would do well to be aware of how to gather chi most effectively, balance it, use it most efficiently, and replenish our ancestral chi if we have diminished it.

The benefits of maximizing our intake of chi and using our chi efficiently are experienced immediately in how we feel. Over the long run, cultivating an abundant supply of chi facilitates enjoying excellent health and vitality well into old age.

My son, Michael, taught me the immediate benefits when he was two. He had a wonderfully happy disposition. Occasionally, however, he would become cranky, unreasonable, and then completely distraught.

One day, I realized that it made no difference whether we did what he wanted or whether he got the toy he wanted. If he was hungry, nothing made him happy until he had something to eat. If he was tired, nothing made him happy until he had a nap. Then, magically, regardless of what he was doing or what toys he had, he was again cheerful as could be.

With this insight, I noticed that I, as an adult, was that way too.

Later on, as an acupuncture practitioner, I observed that when I took care of my chi, particularly when I practiced my T'ai Chi regularly, I rarely got a cold or flu from the many sick people I would treat. If I neglected to care for my chi, the first sick person I saw would bless me with whatever bug they had and I would get sick with it. I experienced this several times, along with three bouts of pneumonia and one of cancer before I accepted the importance of getting sufficient rest, eating wisely, and daily cultivating my chi rather than downing a cup of coffee to perk up and soldier on.

Although taking care of a healthy child's chi is pretty simple—good food and sufficient rest being the main ingredients—these alone are not sufficient for adults.

Replenishing our energy from the food we eat and the air we breathe is relatively easy, but replenishing what we have inherited from our parents, our ancestral chi, is very difficult. This is why a favorable balance between what we take in and what we use is preferable to needlessly expending and prematurely depleting our ancestral chi.

Before examining how we can most efficiently replenish our chi, let's start by having a closer look at how we squander our chi and how we can conserve it.

Chi Burners

With the help of friends at Cultivating Your Chi workshops I have given, I have compiled the following list of some of the common ways of exhausting our chi more rapidly than a balanced life otherwise requires.

- Overwork
- Being tense
- Anger
- Fear
- Grief
- Depression
- Interpersonal conflict
- Disease
- Medications
- Chemotherapy/ Radiation
- Excessive speech
- Getting too cold or too hot

- Refined Sugar
- Drugs
- Extreme exercise
- Lack of sleep
- Coffee/Caffeine
- Excessive alcohol
- Smoking
- Sex (for men)
- Overeating
- Overexertion
- Obsessing
- Worrying

No doubt, you can add to the list. The point is, the root of most of the chi burners listed above is stress. Most of the chi burners are a way to diminish the pain of wanting something other than what is. By burning off some of our chi, we temporarily reduce the internal pressure we feel when we are at odds with what is happening. The root of most of the ways we exhaust our chi is our mind, which becomes attached to an interpretation of reality that we believe to be real, generating a strong effect inside us.

A puritanical view of chi burners is neither realistic nor helpful. For example, the chi consumed by physically processing a strong drink or a cigarette that helps one regain emotional equilibrium after a particularly difficult emotional experience may use much less chi than being deeply upset for days after the event. An occasional glass of wine, delicious dinner topped off with a big dessert, and an after-dinner Scotch followed by sensuous sex will make most people forget about a tough week at work. Fair enough.

On the other hand, a six pack every night or a pack of cigarettes a day is not such a good deal for our chi. Habitual use of our favorite chi burners anesthetizes us and makes it more difficult to sort out what is bothering us. Even worse, as we well know, chronic abuse of chi burners over time will injure us.

When our psyche is confused and at odds with reality, we instinctively are drawn to chi burners that are specific to the aspect of ourselves that is confused and at odds. Understanding how this works and which chi burners go with each aspect of our psyche can be a great help in seeing where we are stuck and clarifying that aspect of ourselves. This knowledge is clearly presented in the Arica *Doors of Compensation*™ training.

Again, viewing chi burners as an evil to avoid misses the point. Life can be hard, and we sometimes become quite upset over things we can do little about. Wise use of the chi burners can help us let go of our emotional attachments, relax, and regain our equilibrium, all of which ultimately minimize the damage from our disagreements with how life is happening and the upset we can feel over it.

As we become more conscious, we can find our equilibrium more easily and diminish the need for habitually and excessively using the chi burners in ways that, over the long run, will cause harm.

Layers of Chi

A simplified but useful way of seeing how the layers of chi inside our bodies are organized is shown in the two diagrams on the following pages, adapted from illustrations in the article "How to Cultivate Your Chi" in the *T'ai Chi Press* by Pat Gorman and Edna Brandt.

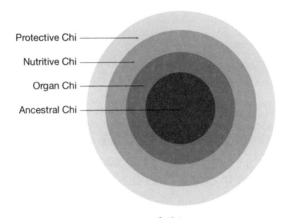

Layers of Chi

The outer layer represents our protective or defensive chi. It is primarily in our skin, hair, adipose tissue, and in general, the outer layer of our body. It keeps us warm or cool as needed and protects us from injury and infection.

The next layer, our nutritive chi, circulates below our skin within the acupuncture meridians, which are like channels of energy carrying chi to each of the internal organs.

The next layer resides in the organs, flesh, and blood.

The deepest layer, in our bone marrow, is our ancestral chi.

Our bodies are intelligent. The outer layer of chi protects the next layer in. The second layer protects the third, which in turn covers and protects our ancestral chi.

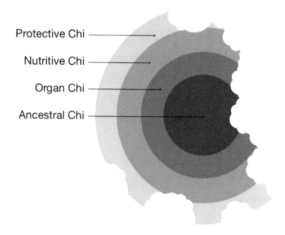

Protective Chi
Nutritive Chi
Organ Chi
Ancestral Chi

Bites Out of Our Chi

When we use up our chi faster than we are replenishing it, it is like taking a bite out of our protective chi. When we take enough bites out to create a weakness in our protective chi, we become vulnerable.

For example, we are more prone to getting a cold or flu after we become overly tired, sleep deprived, or physically cold, particularly if we are also relying on caffeine or other stimulants to propel us onward when we should call it a day. Our body gets sick, takes us out of the game, and says we need a rest.

If we continue to take bites out of our chi, for example, by habitually smoking, sooner or later, we will wear a hole in the meridian layer of our chi. Our lungs will have trouble getting sufficient chi, and we'll begin to have difficulty breathing, a deeper level of illness. Carry on too long, and we chew a hole in our chi so deep that our lungs can no longer repair themselves and become diseased with emphysema or lung cancer.

Long-term use of medications depletes our chi in the organs that are responsible for breaking down and eliminating those medications. It also disturbs the delicate chemical and hormonal balances that are collaterally affected by medications that have a global effect on our whole system. Over time, we develop side effects, which in turn lead to more medications, more side effects, and so on, each further depleting our chi.

Our body, in its wisdom, will replenish the outer layers of chi that become depleted by taking chi from a deeper level to fill in the gaps, but there are limits to what it can do. Continuing to deplete our chi eventually exhausts our deepest level of chi, our ancestral chi. When it is gone, we die.

Learning to balance, conserve, and nourish our chi is essential, particularly if we are dealing with a serious illness such as cancer, where the treatments, while having the potential to save our lives, also consume a lot of our energy.

Chapter 6

Balancing Your Chi

We all have our habitual ways of depleting our chi. Sometimes, we consistently work beyond when we should call it a day. Some are addicted to drugs, alcohol, tobacco, or sugar. Some of us are fond of extreme exercise or excessive sex. Sometimes, we set ourselves up for extreme emotional or physical trauma. Sometimes, we seem to crave emotional drama and spend a lot of energy creating and then dealing with it, again and again.

Each of the chi burners taxes our chi in specific ways, and repeatedly using them imbalances and eventually depletes our chi. We also come into the world with our particular strengths and vulnerabilities, where the inevitable hard knocks of life affect us more than they might someone else. In short, life has a way of taking us out of balance.

The ancient Chinese noticed that the moment our chi is out of balance, our bodies display several distinct signs. Our odor changes. Our emotional responses become either more or less than what one would consider appropriate to what is going on around us. We might be overly fearful or angry, given what is going on in the moment around us. In other words, our emotional response is arising more from what is going on inside of us than what is going on around us.

Our tone of voice changes, and a subtle color shows around our temples. The imbalance is also reflected in our pulses. We have twelve pulses, six of which can be felt on each of our wrists. Each shows the strength and quality of the chi going to its corresponding internal organ.

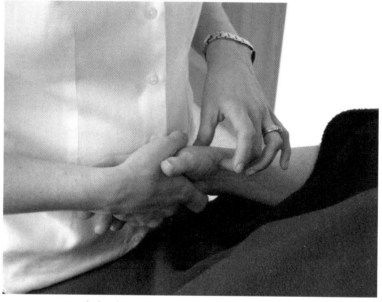

April checking pulses. (Photo by David Goodell.)

By feeling these twelve pulses, a skilled practitioner can determine the strength and quality of the chi going to the heart, small intestines, liver, gall bladder, kidneys, bladder, spleen, stomach, lungs, and colon, plus the two functions responsible for circulation and maintaining temperature. When we are healthy, the twelve pulses are in complete balance. The moment we go out of balance, the imbalance can be felt in our pulses.

These subtle signs—odor, emotion, sound of our voice, color, and pulses—can show a well-trained practitioner of Classical Five Element Acupuncture where our chi has become blocked or depleted long before any disease sets in. The acupuncture points are then used to restore the balanced flow of chi.

Level of the Illness

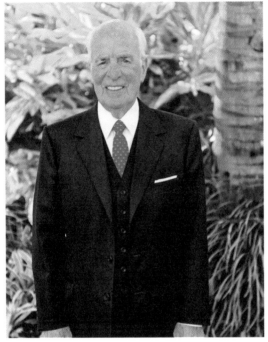

J. R. Worsley. (Photo courtesy of Stephen "Tuna" Flores.)

J. R. Worsley, my acupuncture teacher, once said,

> When the body is sick, the mind worries, and the spirit grieves. When the mind is sick, the body and spirit suffer from its confusion. When the spirit is sick, we lose the will to care for our mind and our body.

If we are going to effectively treat someone who is ill, we also need to pay attention to the level of the illness. We need to know whether it is coming from something that has overwhelmed the person physically or mentally or left them demoralized, frustrated, and resigned. In other words, is the source of trouble on the level of the body or of the mind or of the spirit?

In December of 2001, my wife and I were separated, my son had gone to college, and I was living alone. Although I had a nice acupuncture practice, had wonderful friends in the T'ai Chi, acupuncture, and music communities, and was actively involved in non-profit work, going home to an empty house at the end of the day was hard. I felt isolated, lonely, and discouraged. On the way home from work during rush hour one evening, I had to turn left onto a busy street from a side road. I waited at a stop sign for a long time with cars piling up behind me. Finally, I zipped out.

The next thing I remember was being removed, strapped to a board, from my car through the hatch in the back. I spent ten days in the hospital recovering from a broken pelvis, broken ribs, my spleen and part of my stomach being thrust into my chest cavity through a ruptured diaphragm, internal bleeding, and other lesser injuries.

I needed two major surgeries. For the first several days, I was sedated and tied to the rails on the sides of the bed to prevent me from removing the various tubes and IVs. I was told later that several friends came to visit and that I tried to talk each of them into untying me. My brother Andrew did, but the staff had to tie me up again as I promptly began pulling out IV lines. My friend Roy brought his guitar and played for me. My friend Grace came and sang for me.

Once I was rational enough to be untied, I resolved to get out of the hospital as soon as possible. I could not walk, and for nearly a week, I could not digest anything. Half of an English muffin for breakfast still sat like a lump in my stomach until late afternoon. Frances, my acupuncture practitioner, treated me twice while I was in the hospital. Her treatments started my stomach functioning again.

As soon as I could put my feet on the floor, I began practicing T'ai Chi. Within a couple days, I was hobbling up and down the corridors using a walker, making a point of passing the nursing station each way. I managed to convince my doctors to send me home several days sooner than expected.

Looking back, I realized that when I was waiting for a break in the traffic at that intersection I did not care sufficiently about myself to wait until it was safe to go. I took a chance and impatiently shot out into the street. While my injuries were physical, the unhappy state I was in diminished my willingness to care for myself and led to the accident. The support and encouragement of family and friends who called, wrote, or came to visit while I was in the hospital and once I got home again helped restore my spirit.

The best practitioners of every health care modality I have seen, from the most high-tech western treatments for cancer to those who practice shamanism, treat the spirit as well as the body.

Years earlier, when it was my turn to receive my daily radiation treatment at the hospital after surgery for cancer, I would lie down on the table beneath the radiation machine. The young woman who administered the treatments would adjust my position until I was properly lined up, and then step out into a shielded booth to activate it.

I paid attention to where I was supposed to lie on the table. Over time, I got pretty good at lying down in the right place. Nevertheless, she moved me all around the table every time I went there. One day, after she again moved me all over the table, I said, "Jane, you've moved me all over the place, but I'm exactly where I first started."

She said, "I know, David. How are you going to get better if nobody touches you?" She was caring for my spirit as well as my physical body. Her touch helped put me at ease, and I have never forgotten her wisdom and compassion.

To me what most distinguishes Classical Five Element Acupuncture is that the points, when employed by a compassionate, attentive practitioner, specifically address the needs of the patient's spirit as well as balance the patient's chi. "Spirit Burial Ground" is a point that helps restore a patient's will to live if he or she has become so resigned as to have essentially given up. The "Gate of Hope" can restore a patient's sense of optimism. "Spirit Hall" imparts the feeling of being relaxed and belonging in the here and now. To me, this way of not only balancing one's chi but also of directly helping restore the strength and health of one's spirit makes Classical Five Element Acupuncture without parallel as a system of healing.

As research continuously confirms, the compassion and attention of our health-care providers and the love and companionship of friends and family are indispensable to becoming and remaining healthy. Give this attention when you can, and welcome it when you need it.

Chapter 7

Nourishing Your Chi

Assuming that the flow of chi throughout your system is reasonably balanced and each of your internal organs is able to function effectively, you have two renewable sources of chi. The first is the air you breathe. The second is the food you eat.

The Air You Breathe

For thousands of years, it has been well known that we can improve our vitality and quality of life by consciously improving our breathing. I'm sure everyone has had the experience of stepping outside, taking that first deep breath of fresh morning air, and feeling invigorated. Or of entering a forest and feeling how much vitality the air among the trees provides. Or of smelling the salty sea air near the ocean. The contrast to the smog-filled air of a major city during rush hour is striking. The most obvious way to increase the amount of chi we get from the air we breathe is to breathe clean, fresh air.

You can also significantly increase the amount of chi you absorb from the air you breathe by allowing yourself to relax and breathe slowly and deeply.

You can further improve the quality of your breathing by placing your attention in your t'an tien, located three finger-widths below your navel and about a third of the way into your lower belly. As you breathe in, let your lower belly expand, filling your lungs from the bottom to the top. As you exhale, simply let your belly relax and your lungs empty from the top to the bottom.

This facilitates using your full lung capacity, not just the upper portion that we normally use. The key is to relax and allow this to happen. With a little practice, it can become second nature, replenishing us and producing a feeling of peacefulness as we are reminded that our life comes at the benevolence of the creation.

Meditation practices that focus our attention on the rise and fall of our breath, yogic practices involving breathing, and chanting or singing hymns where we breathe as one, all remind us that we are inseparable from the rest of creation and the life-giving chi it provides all living beings. In fact, the word "spirit" comes from the Latin word "spiritus," meaning "breath." Beyond filling us with vitality and sustaining our life, our breath provides inspiration, clarity, and a sense of intercon-nectedness with something much greater than our individual self—all essential for a healthy life.

Relaxing and breathing clean air slowly and deeply greatly increases the amount of chi we receive and enhances our con-nection with the entire creation.

The Food You Eat

Your digestion begins in your mouth. You will get the most benefit from what you eat (and drink) by following the old adage, "Chew your drink and drink your food." Relax and take your time when you eat, and chew thoroughly. Eating slowly will also give you time to notice when you have had enough and it's time to stop.

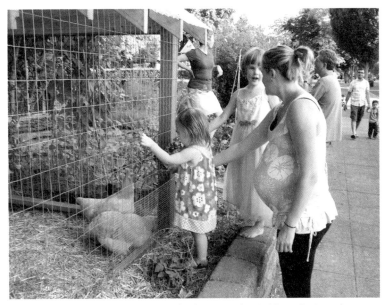

April and Esther's garden, chickens, and neighbors in Seattle.
(Photo by David Goodell.)

You can further increase the amount of chi you receive from your food by eating fresh, local, and in season. Nature, in its wisdom, generally provides the food we need in the time and place we live.

Eskimos in arctic regions, for example, need the many calories that blubber provides. Blubber in Florida would generate way too much warmth inside us for it to be a healthy choice. Likewise, oranges that grow in the tropics have the effect of cooling us off—appropriate in the intense heat of that climate. For people in colder climates, however, citrus fruit and juice can aggravate arthritis.

Fresh food is closer to life and has more chi in it than something that has been frozen or stored in a can. Even those have more chi than something that has been ground up and stored in a box or bag for who knows how long. I am not advocating a diet totally predicated on what grows in your yard in season. I am saying that, in general, you will get more energy from fresh food that nature provides in the vicinity where you live.

Sufficient water is also essential. As a general guide, take your weight in pounds and divide that by two to get the number of fluid ounces of water you need each day. So, for example, if you weigh 120 pounds, you need 60 ounces of water each day. This is in addition to whatever tea, juice, etc. you drink, which your body must digest before absorbing. If you are overweight, the amount recommended above may be too much. Pay attention to how much water feels appropriate for you.

Quality of Our Food

While these simple food recommendations would have been sufficient prior to the Second World War, the industrialization of our world and of agriculture since then has fundamentally altered our lifestyles, the environment, the quality of our air, soil, and water, our food sources, and our food choices with far-reaching consequences for our health.

Airborne mercury, arsenic, and other pollutants from burning coal, as well toxins produced by other industries, now permeate our air, water, soil, and food.

Large-scale farming practices commonly depend on chemical fertilizers to make depleted soil productive. The crops from this soil are deprived of the trace minerals they would receive from balanced, organically enriched soils. Pesticides and herbicides have become mainstays, as have genetically modified crops that tolerate herbicides and pesticides well.

Livestock are often severely confined and sickened with food that is not and never has been their natural diet, which was grown in depleted soils enriched by chemical fertilizers. These sick animals are then given antibiotics to keep them alive and growth hormones to maximize their production of milk, eggs, and meat.

Deprived of the natural variety of plants they would eat if left to range freely, the foods they provide to us are not only seriously deficient of essential vitamins and fatty acids; they also contain toxic chemicals, hormones, antibiotics, and genetically modified proteins.

We eat foods that are out of season where we live, were harvested before they were ripe, and are then shipped thousands of miles to our grocery store. Many were bred to maintain their beautiful appearance over the trip rather than provide optimum nutrition for us. We refine, mill, and bleach our grains. We extract and concentrate sugars and high fructose sweeteners (major contributors to cancer, heart disease, and diabetes), which we consume in unprecedented quantities. To top it off, we add preservatives that change the quality of what we eat and package these foods in wraps and containers, many of which leach toxic chemicals into the food.

Among the more egregious recent forays into alteration of nature's food supply, motivated by the never-ending push for higher profits, is genetically modified crops. There is increasingly strong evidence that genetically modified crops come at a high cost to our health. My friend and fellow T'ai Chi student, Terry Cook, PhD in neuropsychopharmacology and pharmaceutical sciences, has spent more than sixteen years in the biopharmaceutical industry. Terry wrote the following for this book:

> Genetic modification (GM) refers to altering genetic material (DNA). One or more genes are inserted into the crop's genome; these include viral or bacterial genes, "artificial" genes, and antibiotic resistance genes. The inserted gene units re-program the DNA blueprint of the plant to produce cells with completely new properties. Each cell has a finite

amount of energy. If that energy is redirected to do something entirely different from the original program, then the organism will be less nutritious. That is, a cell that is now programmed to make proteins protecting the organism from pesticides will not have the same nutritional value as the natural version.

The dangers of GM foods and food crops are significant and varied, from the introduction of foreign proteins into the food chain to the generation of antibiotic-resistant bacteria. Although GM foods have been available for the past 15 years, their safety for human consumption has never been adequately proven.

There are two primary sources of GM foods: GM ingredients used in processed foods and products from food animals fed GM feed. The FDA does not require any of the GM-containing products to be labeled as such, despite studies showing that animals raised on GM feed ARE different from those raised on non-GM feed and that GM material has been found in the resulting products, including meat, eggs, and milk.

The nutritional value of GM foods is not improved over non-GM foods, and GM foods contain many components that are detrimental to long-term health. For example, the use of rBGH in dairy cattle yields milk that often contains higher levels of pus and bacteria in the milk. This leads to an increased use of antibiotics to combat the infections. The antibiotic residues end up in milk and dairy products. These residues can cause allergic reactions in sensitive individuals and contribute to the growth of antibiotic-resistant bacteria. In addition, research has shown elevated levels of "insulin-like growth factor-1" (IGF-1) in dairy products produced from rBGH-treated cows. These findings are significant because numerous studies now demonstrate that IGF-1 is an important factor in the growth of breast, prostate, and colon cancers.

One of the major health concerns with GM food is its potential to increase allergies in humans eating GM-containing foodstuffs. Without GM labels, consumers are unable to determine which products are free of GM ingredients.

The top four GM food crops produced in the US are soybeans, corn, edible cottonseed, and rapeseed (canola oil), followed by sugar beets and potatoes. Ingredients made from these GM products are ubiquitous in US processed foods. It is now estimated that fully 90 percent of all US processed foods contain genetically modified ingredients, presenting an ever-growing hazard to healthy nutrition.

If the product label lists high fructose corn syrup, corn syrup, corn sugar, soy lecithin, soy, cottonseed oil, or canola oil, it's likely from GM food crops unless otherwise indicated, usually by the label "non-GMO" or "Organic". Soy protein has also been added to increase protein content in fast-food burgers. To ensure your health, read the labels and minimize your intake of processed foods.

It seems we have lost touch with the sources of our nourishment, forgetting that our well-being is dependent on the well-being of the web of life around us.

While we commonly think of food as simply stuff we eat, we would do well to remember that it comes from plants and animals that also have a spirit. The food they provide nourishes our mind and our spirit as well as our physical body. I encourage you to respect and appreciate them. If we treat them well and they are healthy, what they provide will be good for us. If we abuse them, distort them, or take them for granted, what they provide will be considerably less beneficial to us.

Much has been written about how our food supply has been compromised, and with good reason. The cumulative effects of the industrialization of our food sources and the environmental degradation we have produced are inter-related and much more severe than any one of these factors taken alone. Additional information about the food we eat is given in the appendix, and a list of resources is provided at the end of this book.

Return to Your Senses

Although our culture focuses far more attention on intellectual development than sensory awareness, we were born with the ability to see, smell, taste, and feel the effects of the air we breathe and the food we eat. Even if non-GMO, organically grown crops, free-range meat and eggs, and wild fish are not available or affordable for you, with a bit of knowledge, it is a simple matter to use your God-given senses to find clean air and foods that provide you with the most energy and vitality.

Smell a ripe peach and smell a can of peaches. Which makes your mouth water? Taste the strawberries, greens, fruits, and crunchy vegetables picked when ripe the day you buy them at your local farmer's market. Compare them to the ones in the plastic box at your major grocery chain. Organic or not, healthy, colorful, great-smelling whole fruits, vegetables, and other fresh produce provide much more chi. In other words, eat food that excites your senses, as close as possible to the form in which nature provides it.

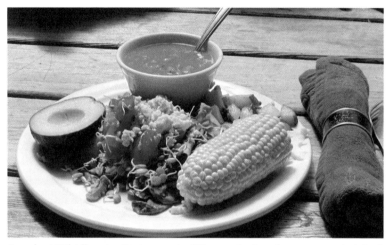

Lunch at Whidbey Institute, most of it organic, locally grown and picked that morning. (Photo by Karen Kohlhaas.)

Regardless of what anyone says you should or shouldn't eat, pay attention to how the foods you eat make you feel. Trust your body. If a particular food doesn't agree with you, don't eat it. If your body feels much better eating something else that you know to be healthy, go for it.

Eating well is more than feeding our physical body with physical food—it is also about nourishing our spirit. Meals can also be a time to enjoy sharing what we have with others, and they with us. Take the time to enjoy the colors, aromas, and flavors of your food and the people with whom you share it. Remember the plants and animals that have given their life so you may have yours.

Chapter 8

Continuum of Health

My friend and colleague, Eliot Ivanhoe, MD, once described a continuum of health ranging from very sick and near death to perfect health with all of one's potential realized. Understanding this continuum provides a useful way of seeing where we are and of being realistic about what we need to feel our best.

What we take to be normal usually is somewhere in the middle of this continuum, considerably less than our optimum state.

If our chi becomes depleted or imbalanced, the first thing we are likely to notice is that we get out of sorts emotionally. We may feel unhappy, frustrated, or afraid. We may have trouble sleeping; we may feel depressed, chronically tired, or get recurring colds, infections, or allergies. If an imbalance worsens, our body will begin to lose its ability to regulate and repair itself.

There are times when a person becomes so ill he or she would die without appropriate medical care. While balancing one's chi is a great help, no matter how ill a person may be, and can be a decisive factor in stabilizing his or her condition and tolerating needed medical care, it is not a substitute for prudent, necessary medical care when a person is seriously ill.

On the other hand, medical treatment for chronic illness may keep us alive, and it may relieve some of the discomfort we feel, but it does not restore perfect health. Long-term use of medications to relieve high blood pressure, depression, asthma, and other symptoms of poor health, while sometimes necessary, further depletes one's chi.

Moving up the continuum of health from chronically feeling poorly to feeling well requires finding and addressing the cause of the patient's poor health rather than just providing a medication that temporarily relieves the symptoms until the medication wears off and the person needs the next dose.

Many factors contribute to causing an illness. There can be physical causes, such as diet, physical activity or lack of it, pathogens, toxins, or allergens. Often, the cause is at a deeper level that has diminished the patient's will to live and to properly care for his or her physical, mental, and spiritual needs. This is why we must also consider the level of the illness, that is, whether it is arising from primarily a physical, emotional, or mental cause. It is rare to feel happy when you feel terrible physically. It is equally difficult to remain physically healthy when you are deeply upset, lacking the will to properly care for yourself, or agonizing about a confusing set of decisions.

In every case I have seen, including physical as well as emotional disease that is treatable but not curable, these factors affect and are affected by the balance and strength of one's chi. For example, the most nutritious meal won't nourish you if your stomach is not getting sufficient energy to digest it. The best supplements won't help a bit if your small intestine is not getting sufficient chi to absorb them. The cleanest diet possible will not prevent your body from becoming polluted if your colon is not getting sufficient chi to eliminate waste or your kidneys are not cleansing your bodily fluids properly. You can breathe the purest air, but it won't help you if your lungs are not receiving enough chi to remain moist, pliable, and able to absorb the oxygen you need.

Each of these functions affects all of the others. Your heart, for example, will not function properly if your whole body is not receiving sufficient oxygen. Your stomach will not digest properly if it is not warm enough. All of your tissues will become weak, including the muscles of your heart and arteries, if your liver does not properly synthesize the necessary proteins from the food your stomach digests, the nutrients your small intestine absorbs, and your circulatory system delivers via the pure clean fluids that comprise your blood when your kidneys are functioning well. Your lungs will not absorb sufficient oxygen and release carbon dioxide if your muscles, lacking adequate nutrition, do not permit your lungs to fill and empty efficiently with each breath.

In short, none of the internal organs can function at its best if even one of the others is not. So, while a medication that strips cholesterol from the patient's system and another that lowers blood pressure may provide temporary help in treating heart disease, for example, you can see the futility of such treatments if the person does not also ensure that all of his or her internal organs are receiving the energy they need to do their jobs properly.

Resolving unhappiness at home or at work—the feeling that one is missing his or her higher calling, feeling isolated or alone, and so on—is often an essential part of healing from any illness, whether physical, mental, or emotional. One of the problems with giving anti-depressants is that they mask how a person feels, making it more difficult for him or her to recognize and address the reason for the unhappiness.

We are amazingly resilient beings. Furthermore, our bodies are completely committed to becoming and remaining well. Once each of our internal organs is getting what it needs to function as nature intended, we have the best possibility of becoming well physically, mentally, and emotionally.

Taking care of one's chi is, therefore, the best way I know to enhance the effectiveness of medical care and open the way to healing even serious chronic illness. It is the only path I know for advancing towards perfect health, with all of one's potential realized.

Types of Acupuncture

There are many types of acupuncture. Some types of acupuncture can be used as anesthesia for patients who cannot tolerate chemical anesthesia. Others use standardized formulas of acupuncture points for treating addictions.

Still others rely on specific combinations of acupuncture points to relieve pain or alleviate symptoms of illness with only minimal attention towards addressing the fundamental imbalance within a particular patient that is preventing an injury from healing or causing his or her illness. While relieving pain and uncomfortable symptoms of illness or addictions is a laudable aim of any health care, there is a serious downside in treating symptoms without attending to the actual cause. It is a bit like, as J. R. Worsley used to say, disconnecting the warning light when your car is low on oil and then continuing on as though the problem has been solved. Symptoms that seemed to be easily relieved at first are likely to become deeper, more serious, and more difficult to heal a bit further down the road.

Classical Five Element Acupuncture is at the other end of the spectrum, focused primarily on helping the person's chi regain its strength and balance. Rather than treat the manifestation of the imbalance, it can help people regain their balance and, with it, their natural ability to heal, regardless of whether they have cancer, heart disease, depression, or any other disease process to which we in the West attach a label.

This type of acupuncture can be enormously helpful when a person is seriously ill. Overcoming injury or illness while one's chi is blocked or out of balance is much more difficult, if not impossible. Becoming well again is also difficult, if not impossible, without addressing the level of the illness and helping the patient regain his or her sense of optimism and enthusiasm for life.

Classical Five Element Acupuncture also excels as preventive care since it can be used to detect and correct imbalances before an illness develops. It can help one breathe well and have optimal digestion, absorption, circulation, elimination, sleep, and so on. These help replenish and use one's chi more efficiently. It can help a person regain his or her mental clarity, joy of life, and with it, the ability and willingness to properly care for him- or herself.

This is why, as a patient's energy comes into balance, he or she commonly feels much better than before the illness. In other words, the person has progressed beyond where he or she started on the continuum of health towards optimum health.

Unfortunately, even the best Classical Five Element Acupuncture, by itself, does not directly replenish ancestral chi, nor does it take us the last leg of the journey to feeling our best.

Stages of Treatment

Most of us seek help when we are sick and unable to get better on our own. We want someone who knows what he or she is doing to fix the problem for us. I certainly did. I used to get severe hay fever. I tried everything I could think of with little success. I did not know how to make it better, and I just wanted someone to make it to go away.

After wanting someone else to fix the illness we are experiencing, as one would like our car mechanic to fix our car, the patients who will experience the most improvement and gain the most lasting benefit go through some additional stages.

The first is realizing that the physical and emotional pain and illness we are experiencing is a way that our body, mind, and spirit call our attention to the lack of balance in our life. It is an opportunity to examine how we relate to our work, family, friends, and society, as well as how we take care of our physical needs. Putting aside social expectations and norms, what is needed to bring the way we live into a better balance that helps each of us, as a unique individual, follow our path in life?

The second is realizing that remaining well is much easier with regular preventative care. Seasonal treatment with Classical Five Element Acupuncture, once one is well, is a great help in staying well.

The third stage is realizing, especially once we pass our mid-thirties, that our bodies no longer regenerate themselves as they once did. A daily practice of cultivating one's chi is indispensable.

Towards Optimum Health

Advancing closer toward optimum health requires our active participation in a daily practice of cultivating our chi, grounded in the natural laws of how our chi works. T'ai Chi, Qi Gong, meditation, and yoga are among the arts that provide a means of becoming more aware of one's essential, timeless nature and of cultivating one's chi.

The elegant, graceful movements of T'ai Chi gather and then circulate our chi without interruption through each of the internal organs in the correct order. Ten minutes of practice in the morning sets the pattern for how we live that day. In the evening, it helps us let go of whatever tensions we have collected and restores order to our system before we head off to bed. Feeling more energetic and enjoying greater clarity, peace, and sense of purpose from an enjoyable, relaxed daily practice becomes a powerful incentive to persevere.

Professor Cheng used to say, "Three things are necessary for success in studying T'ai Chi: perseverance, natural ability, and correct teaching. Of these, correct teaching is the most important. Without it, no amount of practice will bring you the full benefit. Natural ability is the least important because, whether success requires practicing a few times or a hundred, in the end it is the same."

It is beyond the scope of this book to provide correct teaching in T'ai Chi. Videos and books can help but are poor second bests to learning from a teacher who understands the art and can guide the student. Nevertheless, if I could offer one word of advice to help you cultivate your chi, it would be "relax." If I could offer a few more, they would be "breathe slowly and deeply into your t'an tien."

Thoughts on Dying

When I was young, my own death seemed too distant to think much about. I thought about it briefly while considering some of my more hazardous adventures and when people I knew passed away, but that was about it.

For those fortunate to live a long life, it seems more natural and more common to prepare for death ahead of time. Regardless of our age, being diagnosed with a life-threatening illness has a way of bringing our attention to our eventual death.

I vividly remember how I felt when I was diagnosed with cancer and realized that I could die soon. Over the years, I also have treated many patients with life-threatening illnesses, some of whom died. I feel I have enough experience on the subject to share some observations and thoughts about it.

My first observation is that facing death is a sobering experience. It has a way of immediately reordering one's priorities. The following questions often come up:

Will I be able to regain my health?

What is the course of this illness and how will I feel?

What will treatment be like? Will it be painful?

How am I going to afford treatment? What if I can't work? How will I live? How can I get the help I will need?

What will happen to family and friends who depend on me? Have I made my intentions clear and my affairs easy to complete for those I will leave behind?

Finally, what will death be like? How can I best prepare myself for what I will experience?

The most helpful thing I have seen for those whose death is approaching is accepting their situation and relaxing. Dying is as natural and healthy a part of life as being born. Fear of what will happen seems to be one of the main obstacles to relaxing and accepting death as a natural part of life.

I deeply appreciate being present when my close friend Tom died and years later when my father died. Their struggle to stay alive was very hard for them, but at a certain point, both relaxed noticeably. Their breathing slowed and softened. With a small sigh, each simply let go. It resembled watching a child finally let go of the day and drift off to sleep.

In contemplating your death, I encourage you to accept your feelings about it without judging them or yourself for having them. I encourage you to make your peace with anyone you have not. Sharing your feelings with someone you trust is an honor and a blessing for that person. It can help the other more fully appreciate life and accept his or her own death when it is time.

For those listening to someone share his or her feelings, I encourage you simply to listen. There is no need to try to change what the other person is feeling, offer false encouragement, and so on. Fear, anger, sadness, a need for understanding, and grief are all part of life and can teach us a lot about compassion and an appreciation for our life and those we love. Your complete attention and willingness to be at ease in the presence of someone facing their death is immensely helpful and comforting.

I have come to see death as beautiful a part of life as birth. Pure spirit enters our body at birth and leaves at death. Death can remind those who are present that our essential self is pure spirit.

I love the Pierre Teilhard de Chardin saying, "We are not human beings having a spiritual experience. We are spiritual beings having a human experience."

Chapter 9

Relax

The essence of conserving your chi is being relaxed.

In 1990, at the age of thirty-eight, I noticed a sore spot under the skin in my neck, a couple inches above and to the right of my Adam's apple. Within a couple weeks, it had grown to the size of a grape. A visit to my doctor quickly led to a biopsy and a diagnosis of squamous cell cancer in a brachial cleft cyst.

I was terrified. I did not feel like eating, and I could not sleep. I felt as if I was burning up inside.

So much for the faith I had placed in my youth, acupuncture treatments, meditating, eating a healthy diet, and practicing my T'ai Chi every (well, almost every) morning upon arising and evening before bed. I believed these things assured me of a long and healthy life. Instead, I had cancer. I could die from it.

After three days, it dawned on me that my timeless essential being was going to remain unchanged regardless of what happened. I felt a wave of peacefulness, which made it possible to sleep well again and, from a clear and rested place, deal effectively with my situation.

The western medical people who took care of me were superb—kind, compassionate, well organized, and skillful. A large portion of my neck was removed.

For nearly two months after surgery, I went to the hospital and received radiation treatments five days a week. After each treatment, I felt like a balloon someone had rubbed on a wool sweater, filled with static electricity. It was an odd and unsettling feeling. So, each day when I got home, I practiced T'ai Chi. After practicing for about fifteen minutes, I would feel tired but steady inside.

Fatigue from radiation treatment is cumulative. By the time my seven-week treatment regimen was finished, my vitality was noticeably diminished. I worked half days treating patients and then went home to rest. My T'ai Chi practice and weekly acupuncture treatments helped a lot, but it still took a year for me to feel my usual zip again.

It was a valuable experience. My arrogant attitude that "if people took care of themselves as I do, they would not get sick" was replaced by a much more humble, compassionate, and realistic understanding. Sage or sinner, sooner or later, we all will die. Sometimes, for reasons we may not fully understand, it seems that people get sick and die before their time.

Blaming ourselves or others when they get sick is not helpful. It sets the stage for feeling resentful at the unfairness of it, remorseful that we didn't live differently, or angry with others because they did not heed our advice and live differently. The end result is more tension and more energy wasted.

The main way we conserve our chi is to relax. I am not talking about spacing out with marijuana or a couple of beers, nor do I mean ignoring the things in our life that need attention, pretending they don't. I mean learning to be relaxed as our regular state, whether we are working, resting, on our way to an appointment, doing errands, facing illness, etc. Everything we do, including dealing with our most difficult personal challenges, is improved by a relaxed approach.

Easier Said Than Done

It is easy to say, "Relax." In reality, relaxing is among the most difficult things to do.

First, our mind insists that there will be grave consequences if we don't accomplish certain things. There are things we must do to live, but the tension we feel around the things we feel concerned about, problems we feel we must solve, and issues we must resolve is a product of our mind. All of the tension we feel boils down to some kind of fear.

Second, this fear not only resides in our mind; it also manifests in our body as stiffness, muscular tension, and eventually disease. Tension in our mind immediately manifests as tension in our body. Just notice how you feel inside the next time you are really angry. The muscles in your face contract and show your anger, no matter how hard you try to conceal it. Your facial muscles are not alone in clenching when you are angry. Your arteries, heart, lungs, and the rest of your body clench too.

The ancient sages looked at a young child and saw someone who was soft and pliable, yet had great stamina, vitality, and a long life ahead. They observed that the ultimate in stiffness is rigor mortis. They would say, "Would you rather be soft, pliable, and full of life—or stiff, hard, and dead?"

This is why Patrick Watson, the founder of the School of T'ai Chi Chuan, helped coin the phrase "strength through softness," and the koan "Why does the tongue outlast the teeth?" To cultivate softness and relaxation is to become more alive. It is also to become more aware because, when we become tense in one part of our body, we generally become less aware of that part of our body.

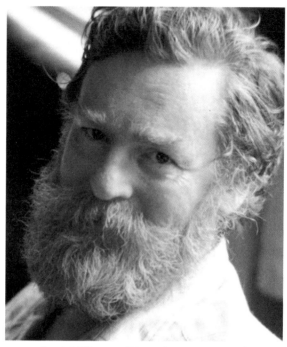

Patrick Watson. (Photo by Pat Gorman.)

We tend to think a healthy body is one with firm abs and taut, sculpted muscles. How contrary to nature! Strength is the difference between how relaxed one set of muscles is and the ability of the opposing set of muscles to contract. Otherwise, our muscles are simply pulling against each other, consuming our energy, blocking the free flow of blood and chi, and aside from satisfying one's vanity, accomplishing nothing.

After studying, practicing and teaching T'ai Chi for thirty some years, I am still struck by how soft and pliable my teachers' bodies are compared to how tense a beginning student's body is and by how much longer an advanced student can practice without tiring compared to the beginner.

Some of the accumulated tensions in our bodies from injuries and old patterns of posture and movement will take a long time to release through our T'ai Chi or yoga practice.

Some may be beyond our ability to release on our own. Many gentle and effective therapies are now available to help release these tensions, including massage, non-force directional chiropractic, zero-balancing, cranio-sacral work, reflexology, and Rolfing, to name a few. Each has its particular virtues, and each addresses specific troubles with our musculoskeletal system in a particular way.

Having experienced many of these, I have noticed that the key determinant to the success of these therapies is the ability of both the practitioner and the patient to be present and focused while working. The better the practitioner's ability to accurately feel where the patient's muscles and ligaments are clenched and gently bring the patient's attention to those stuck places so that the patient can consciously relax them, the more effective the therapy will be. In the end, it is the patient who must become aware of where and how he or she is holding tensions and consciously let those tensions relax.

The main reason parts of our body get stuck is because our bodies are storing pain in those places. When someone touches them, they help bring our attention to this pain, and we feel it. If practitioners listen well, they can read our ability to relax and let the pain and stiffness dissolve. They will feel our body relax, which will allow them to go deeper into the painful areas. They will feel the moment our body resists and know they need to lighten their touch and give us more time to let the area relax. Trying to force or hurry the process generally results in our body further tensing up to resist the intrusion.

Breathing slowly and deeply while someone is working on our body facilitates relaxing our stuck places. As we relax, our breathing will naturally continue to slow and deepen, further helping us relax and advance towards greater awareness and health.

Interestingly, I have found that memories of physical and emotional traumas have often surfaced as I have released the tensions in my body. In addition to easing physical pain, relaxing stuck or painful areas helps release past emotional hurts and the energy it takes to "brace ourselves" from re-experiencing such a trauma. Again, our body, our mind, and our spirit are interconnected. Their well-being manifests in our level of awareness.

As we become more relaxed, we become softer. Our chi flows more easily, and we become more resilient emotionally and physically. Our real strength and vitality returns along with our emotional resilience. We become more able to go with the flow and avoid getting injured again. Our immunity and ability to heal from disease and injury of every kind is greatly improved. As we become softer, we also become more relaxed.

The legendary Yang Cheng Fu, a member of the Yang family and Professor Cheng's T'ai Chi teacher, was a peerless martial artist. Professor Cheng said that the arms of his teacher, Yang Cheng Fu, were several times heavier than those of a normal person because the accumulation of chi through his constant T'ai Chi practice had made his bones extraordinarily dense and hard. He also said Yang Cheng Fu's muscles were so relaxed and soft that his arms felt like steel wrapped in cotton. Yang Cheng Fu's body was completely alert, sensitive, and able to move in harmony with his surroundings without fear and the attendant muscular tension.

The special benefit of T'ai Chi is cultivating the ability to move through life in a relaxed, balanced, and conscious way. Our morning practice establishes the principles that will carry us through the day—standing aligned with gravity so our bones hold us up and our muscles can relax, breathing slowly and deeply, eyes relaxed, and attention centered in our t'an tien. Practicing again before bed gives us the space to let go of the tensions and concerns of the day, balance our energy, and sleep more peacefully.

As you will quickly discover if you take up T'ai Chi, becoming softer and more relaxed is not the same as becoming weak.

On the contrary, your legs will become much stronger, your balance steadier, and your stamina greatly improved.

As we become softer, we also become less fearful and more conscious. The best antidote to getting injured and accumulating tension from physical as well as emotional encounters is a relaxed, awake state that enables us to live in harmony with our surroundings and those around us. This is the essence of T'ai Chi and why the closing move in the T'ai Chi form is called "Entering the Tao."

Chapter 10

Cultivating Your Chi

Although our food and the air we breathe provide the easy ways of nourishing our chi, these alone do not replenish our ancestral chi without additional effort on our part. Furthermore, while exercise is generally beneficial, most exercise, no matter how much exertion is involved, makes little if any contribution towards replenishing your ancestral chi. Cultivating your chi, and especially replenishing your ancestral chi, only happens from a consistent, daily practice following specific principles.

In speaking of cultivating one's chi, Lao Tzu, the great Chinese sage, wrote:

> This is why the sage governs himself by
>> Relaxing the mind
>> Reinforcing the abdomen
>> Gentling the will and
>> Strengthening the bones. [1]

By "relaxing the mind," we diminish the energy we consume by thinking and experiencing the emotions our thoughts produce.

"Reinforcing the abdomen" is not about eating a lot and growing a big belly, nor is it about getting rock-hard abs. It is about developing the habit of breathing slowly and deeply and welcoming the chi of heaven into our lower belly, an area also known as the "Sea of Chi."

"Gentling the will" refers to knowing moderation, i.e., when to rest rather than continue pursuing our goal, regardless of how exhausted we may feel.

"Strengthening the bones" refers to replenishing our ancestral chi, which is stored in our bone marrow and kidneys.

Strengthening the bones is actual, not just a figure of speech. My friend and one of my T'ai Chi teachers, Margaret Matsumoto, had a bone density scan done as part of her physical exam when she turned sixty. Her legs and hips showed the same bone density as a healthy thirty-year-old.

How can we follow Lao Tzu's advice? In T'ai Chi, following an ancient Taoist teaching previously mentioned on page 35 and 36, we begin by placing our attention in our t'an tien, a point three-fingers-width below our navel and about one third of the way in. At first this may seem absurd, a boring waste of time. It can also feel downright frustrating as our mind constantly wanders off to thoughts that seem more entertaining or more pressing.

Take heart and persevere. When your mind wanders, bring your attention back to your t'an tien. Just as with practice you learned to ride a bike, with practice you can learn to recognize your many thoughts as simply the chatter of your mind and bring your attention back to your t'an tien. Gradually, your attention will spend more time focused in your t'an tien.

Next, lightly touch the roof of your mouth where the hard and soft palate meet with the tip of your tongue and keep it there. Then, as you inhale, imagine your breath is filling your t'an tien. You may need to loosen any tight clothing around your middle so that your belly can expand as you inhale. Breathing into the t'an tien has the effect of drawing our diaphragm, the large dome-shaped muscle that separates our chest cavity from our abdominal cavity, downward towards the t'an tien. This fills our lungs from the bottom to the top, as we would a pitcher of water. As we exhale, the diaphragm relaxes, and our lungs empty from the top to the bottom, again as water would pour out of the pitcher.

This uses much more of our lung capacity than our usual shallow, upper chest breathing. It gives us more energy, and it is deeply relaxing.

Finally, as you inhale slowly and deeply into your t'an tien, imagine a point of light starting at the tip of your coccyx, or tailbone, and traveling up your spine to the top of your head. As you exhale slowly, imagine the point of light traveling down the front of your body along the midline. It starts down the front of your head to the roof of your mouth, crosses down through the tip of your tongue, continues down to your solar plexus, then to your t'an tien, and then finally finishes at your perineum, on the bottom of your trunk. Continue this pattern with each breath.

Our lower belly contains the greater omentum, a sheet of connective tissue that surrounds, supports, and protects our internal abdominal organs. Focusing our attention in our t'an tien deepens our breathing and collects our chi in our lower belly among the folds of the omentum. Furthermore, the heat generated by our mind's attention in the t'an tien warms the fluids of our lower belly, causing the chi that accumulates there to overflow and then travel up your spine in one of the two deepest acupuncture meridians that nourish all of the meridians traveling to each of the internal organs. A beautifully clear explanation of this is given by Professor Cheng in *Cheng Tzu's Thirteen Treatises on T'ai Chi Ch'uan*, listed in the Resources section at the end of this book.

Imagining the point of light traveling down the front as you exhale brings the energy we normally waste with our chattering mind down toward our t'an tien along the second of the two deepest meridians. It then gathers the energy we normally waste by the various strong emotions we experience in our chest, or emotional center, and brings this energy back to our t'an tien as well. As more energy accumulates in the t'an tien, more energy becomes available to nourish all of the internal organs.

As you practice, welcome the breath into your t'an tien. Over time, it will become your normal way of breathing.

The value of breathing slowly and deeply into the t'an tien is enormous. The following story illustrates its importance.

After becoming deeply exhausted by a demanding workload, my friend, colleague, and T'ai Chi teacher, Pat Gorman, developed a severe form of hemolytic anemia, an autoimmune disorder where her white cells began attacking her red cells. Those with her genetic profile who survive the first month of this illness often die within two years. It is unusual for someone to survive beyond five.

Although Pat has suffered greatly from this illness and complications brought on by it, she has nevertheless remained not only alive but also very productive as an acupuncturist, teacher, artist, and writer for over seventeen years.

She recently completed the task of interviewing Professor Cheng's former patients, many of whom had overcome life-threatening illnesses, to see which movements derived from the T'ai Chi form he had assigned to them to help them regain their health. Pat has reconstructed and presented this knowledge via the T'ai Chi Foundation in a DVD entitled *Roots and Branches Five Element Qi Gong*.

Five years ago, Pat contracted Legionnaire's Pneumonia and slipped into unconsciousness. She emerged two weeks later to see a doctor standing over her. His only words were, "Blink once if you want to live. Blink twice if you want us to let you go."

Pat had no idea what had happened to her, where she was, who he was, or what he was talking about. She blinked several times in astonishment. He turned off the respirator. Fortunately, Pat managed to take a breath, then another, and continue on. She did not, however, have sufficient strength even to move a finger. So, she practiced the only thing she could—breathing into her t'an tien. After a time, while she continued this slow, deep breathing, she imagined that she was practicing the T'ai Chi form. Over a period of several months, her strength gradually returned.

Pat is an inspiration to me, and a joy to be around. While the excellent medical care she has received saved her life more than once, she credits living so long with this illness and her remarkable accomplishments to her strong will, acupuncture treatments, and her practice of Qi Gong and T'ai Chi.

No matter how sick you may be, I encourage you to be patient and persevere, breathing slowly and deeply into your t'an tien.

Perseverance

Although I have seen many instances of patients feeling much better soon after starting acupuncture treatment, beginning their T'ai Chi practice, changing their diet, and so on, more often progress is gradual. This is especially true with serious illness that has been going on for some time. It is important to remember that by the time we have become seriously ill, we have been out of balance for quite some time. Nature is kind—it gives us several increasingly strong warnings before we become seriously ill. The first signs—our color, sound, odor, emotion, and pulses—tend to go unnoticed. A well-trained practitioner of Classical Five Element Acupuncture often can pick them up, but many times, we cannot see them ourselves.

As an imbalance worsens, the signs of distress become more noticeable. We may lack our usual vitality, we may get frequent colds or infections, our appetite and sleep may be off, and we may feel ill at ease. It is very common for those with cancer, for example, to say that they felt tired and stressed out for a year before being diagnosed. If we have missed or had no means of dealing with the more gentle signs of distress nature provided, the time comes when nature within us finally can no longer keep it together, and we become seriously ill.

Being very sick is uncomfortable and frightening. It is normal to want or even become desperate for an immediate solution. While strong interventions may be necessary, a true process of healing takes longer and requires perseverance.

Becoming well again is a bit like restoring a neglected garden. Debris needs to be cleared, weeds need to be pulled, the soil turned, and organic matter worked into the soil and given time to enrich it. Then you can plant your seeds. They sprout and grow at their own pace as you continue to tend the garden, watering, weeding, enriching, and turning the soil as needed. As J. R. Worsley used to say, "You cannot plant your corn on Monday and expect to harvest it on Tuesday." Nor does it do any good to become impatient and pull on the shoots to hasten their growth. Nature, in its time, will give you a plentiful harvest if you are willing to invest the effort, care, and patience to help it along.

Acupuncture treatment will help facilitate the healing process, but it can take time for our body, mind, and spirit to heal. Changing one's food choices and habits will take some effort. Learning T'ai Chi definitely takes patience and perseverance. One must practice daily to experience the full benefit that is possible.

We live in a culture that expects instant results, but nature does not work that way. Professor Cheng's experience overcoming tuberculosis is a great illustration. Pat Gorman's recovery from Legionnaire's pneumonia is another. It took me a year of daily T'ai Chi practice to regain my vitality from seven weeks of radiation. Considering the alternatives in each of those examples, a consistent daily practice of cultivating our chi changed the trajectory of our health from approaching death to achieving our best possible health—a bargain by any measure.

I cannot encourage you enough to invest the necessary time and effort. Not only will you maximize your chances of escaping serious and unpleasant illness; you will also feel much better than you did before you got sick in the first place. A lifetime of perseverance will produce a lifetime of benefit.

Best of all, it is enjoyable, and it feels good.

Chapter Notes

[1] Cheng Man-jan, "Lao-Tzu: 'My words are very easy to understand.'" Lectures on the Tao Teh Ching.

Chapter 11

Consciousness

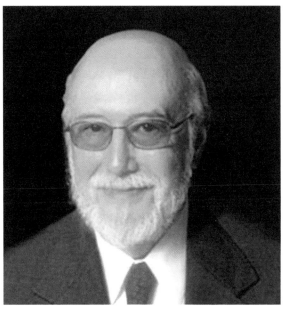

Oscar Ichazo. (Photo courtesy of Arica Institute.)

Oscar Ichazo said, "Consciousness is that which recognizes itself."™ [1] It is awareness. It has no other components. Gautama the Buddha said, "Find what has not been born, because what has not been born will never disappear."[2]

In other words, look around you. Everything you see will change. Our bodies will mature, age, and die. Our ideas change and evolve over time. Many of the things I once took to be true I now see are not. Our feelings change. We can become very angry with someone, and a little while later, all is forgiven, and we love that person. Our thoughts, feelings, and every physical object you can see, including your body, sooner or later will change.

Seek that which doesn't change.

The more aware we become of the aspect of us that is timeless, that has never been born, the more the fear at the root of all of our tensions can begin to dissolve. With greater awareness comes a greater ability to relax. The more relaxed we are, the less we are preoccupied. The less preoccupied we are, the more clearly we see our place in the world as it is—accurately and without preconceptions. The more clearly we understand our place in the world, the more realistic we become. The more realistic we become, the more secure we feel.

Our mind has three aspects.

The first is the right hemisphere of our brain, which collates the vast amount of energetic information we continually receive via our senses and gives us an awareness of the present moment: what it feels like, smells like, looks like, sounds like, and so on. This awareness makes us feel connected with each other and everything around us. We feel at one with the entire creation.

The second is the left hemisphere of our brain, which selects a small portion of that information, filters out the rest, and draws conclusions from what it has taken in. This aspect of our mind conceptualizes a past, present, and future. It gives us linear thinking: the ability to compare, reason, plan, communicate, and interact with each other and our environment.

The third aspect of our mind is simply awareness. It has no thoughts, no components.

Jill Bolte Taylor, a brain researcher at Harvard, suffered a massive stroke in the left hemisphere of her brain and later wrote about it in her book, *My Stroke of Insight*. She also gave a fascinating talk about it on the TED.org website. She described losing the functions of the left hemisphere of her brain one by one: the ability to reason, dial the phone, speak, and then move. She further described becoming much more aware of the functioning of the right hemisphere of her brain, which continued having a beautiful experience of feeling connected with everything around her, free of any worry or concern.

The third aspect of her mind, simple awareness, was simultaneously observing the entire experience, like a perfect witness.

Another of the Arica Axioms is, "Our consciousness can be awake or asleep."™ [3] When our consciousness is awake, we are aware of the timeless aspect of our self, simple awareness. When our consciousness is asleep we believe the temporary aspects of our self—our thoughts, feelings, identity in the world, even our bodies—are the real us.

All of these temporary aspects of our self will end when we die. To the extent we believe those temporary aspects of ourselves to be who we are, we forget the aspect of us that is timeless. We miss the opportunity to relax and live in harmony with the Tao.

Experience has taught me that missing the opportunity to relax and live in harmony with the Tao is the major cause of illness.

I wish it were a simple matter of grasping this concept for our consciousness to become and remain fully awake. My experience is that this awareness comes and goes. Meditation and T'ai Chi are among the ways to awaken and gradually stabilize this awareness of our essential, timeless nature.

The more aware we become, the less physical and emotional tension we experience and the more we are able to relax and cultivate our chi.

Chapter Notes

[1] Oscar Ichazo, *The Human Process for Enlightenment and Freedom* (New York: Arica Institute, 1976), 74.

[2] Oscar Ichazo, *The Human Process for Enlightenment and Freedom* (New York: Arica Institute, 1976), 67.

[3] Copyrighted Arica Axiom, by Oscar Ichazo.

Chapter 12

Living in Harmony

The Tao functions according to natural laws. Everything has its timing and its cycles. We do not make these up, and we cannot change them. Learning them is the basis of science and of following the Tao.

The ancient sages were keen observers of nature. They understood and lived according to principles and natural cycles that we tend to overlook. Just as we suffer if we ignore gravity and jump from too high a place, we also suffer from our lack of understanding and willingness to live in harmony with these natural laws and cycles.

The fundamental cycles of yin and yang include night and day, the seasons, and even our lifetime. The cycle of yin and yang can be seen with more clarity across the five phases, or elements, and across the seasons. Each season makes an essential contribution in the cycle of life. It is very easy to see if you have a garden or spend some time outdoors.

Here in Seattle, the winter rain replenishes the ground water, and snow accumulates in the mountains, providing the snowpack that feeds the streams and rivers through the rest of the year. Plants grow, but very slowly. It is almost as if they are all resting, waiting for the increasing light and heat of spring to take off.

As spring approaches, tiny shoots appear, buds show on our fruit trees, and we can feel the energy of the season change. A tremendous burst of new growth comes as we get more light and warmth.

Summer finally arrives with a definite feeling of warmth and light. The days are long, tomatoes set their fruit, peas, raspberries, and cherries ripen. People wear shorts, and the park is filled with children playing and parents conversing until bedtime. It feels good to have the windows open and feel the breeze. The sun and warmth are deeply relaxing.

Another change comes toward the end of August. You can hear it, see it, feel it, and you can smell it. The hot parched smell of dry grass changes to a softer fragrance as the air cools and things ripen. The light starts to turn more of a golden hue, and the sounds outside start to mellow. It is late summer. More fruits and vegetables ripen. It's time to gather them and put some aside for the coming winter.

The most obvious sign of autumn, the next season, is the changing leaves. We see trace minerals on full display as trees prepare to let go of foliage that has served its purpose. Leaves fall to the ground and enrich the soil. We gather the last of the garden plants, chop them up, and put them in the compost bin with manure from our chickens to hasten their composting into the rich soil that later goes on our garden. We plant a cover crop to fix nitrogen in the soil. The cover crop will sprout and then seem dormant over the winter. When early spring comes, the cover crop grows rapidly, enriching the soil further.

Although each season invariably follows the one before, we get rain in the summer, there are hot days in the spring, and some things, like our cover crop, sprout in autumn. In fact, each season has all five phases or elements within it.

The cycle of these five elements also goes on inside us continuously. Living in harmony with the natural cycles of the seasons and times of day is essential if we want to flourish.

Planting at the wrong time of year, failing to provide water over the hot summer, or waiting too long to gather your crop will yield a meager harvest. Similarly, life without a sense of timing and proportion will produce less than it could.

I encourage you to experiment a bit. In the winter, when the days are shorter and the nights are long, try going to bed earlier and sleeping later. The rest of nature is resting and gathering its strength. Why not us?

Spring is a great time to hatch the new ideas you've contemplated over the relative rest of winter. Be realistic about which ideas you wish to implement, about what is actually possible. Not every flower can produce a fruit.

Summer, when the days are long and the nights are short, is the time to get up early and work longer to bring your plans to fruition. Be sure to spend time with your friends and family. Having some fun is important, giving you memories to warm your heart over the winter.

Gather your harvest as it ripens in the late summer, and be thankful for it.

Let the crisp air and splendor of fall colors remind you of your perfect, timeless nature in an impermanent body. Follow nature's lead as you let go of what has served its purpose and is no longer needed.

Electric lights and a fixed work schedule detach us from this natural cycle. We would do well to remember it and live in harmony with it. We are part of it, and it goes on within as well as outside of us.

Each of the five elements within us receives more energy during its season, and less during the other seasons. If we are out of balance, we tend to feel our best when the extra energy of that season mitigates our imbalance, and not so well during another that exacerbates it.

The Twelve Officials

The ancient sages recognized that the internal organs have more than a physical job. In addition to their physical duties, each has mental and emotional responsibilities that determine our physical health, clarity of mind, and the quality of life that we experience. We experience this quality of life with what the ancient sages referred to as our spirit, which gives purpose and meaning to everything we do.

The ancients recognized that our intelligence, our emotions, and our deepest knowing are much more than the product of our brain. They come from our whole body functioning in a balanced way. So, the ancient sages referred to the ten major internal organs and two additional functions as the twelve "officials."

Each of the twelve officials belongs to one of the elements. Following are very brief descriptions of the officials, listed according to their element and their season of peak energy.

Water Element
Winter

The Bladder official provides sufficient fluids for every part of our body. Too little and the officials become parched; too much and they become water logged. Healthy functioning of this official also gives our body, mind, and spirit the fluidity needed to adapt and persevere.

The Kidney official cleanses the fluids in our body, sees to their proper distribution, and is the storehouse of our ancestral chi. It provides the will and stamina for our body, mind and spirit.

Wood Element
Spring

The Liver official, or "Great Planner," determines our master plan. Physically, it knows what proteins to synthesize so our body can grow, function, and repair itself properly. Mentally and emotionally, it provides us with the vision needed to see our path in life.

The Gall Bladder official is the great "Decision Maker." Physically, this official decides when to release its bile to facilitate the digestion of fats. Mentally and emotionally, it makes the appropriate decisions and provides the sense of timing that allows us to implement our plans.

Fire Element
Summer

The Heart official, or "Supreme Controller," not only pumps our blood. It also is the seat of the Divine within each of us. Like a wise, benevolent emperor, providing for the needs of the entire kingdom of body, mind, and spirit, it relies on insight and understanding. It makes sure the needs of all of the officials are met. It leads with steadiness, compassion, and courage. In the opening move of the T'ai Chi sword form, the right index and middle fingers touch the heart and then point forward. It is called "Divinity Leads the Way."

The Small Intestine, or "Sorter of the Pure from the Impure," is the closest companion of the heart. The sorter knows what is good for our body, mind, and spirit and what is not. On a physical level, every food has some components that are good and some that are useless or even toxic. This official discriminates, absorbs what is useful, and then lets the rest go by.

Our "Heart Protector" governs our circulatory system and also has the function of protecting our heart. The Heart Protector does not have a specific organ associated with it. However, the pericardium (the membrane that surrounds and protects the heart), the blood vessels, and our sexual organs are ruled by this official. When functioning properly, our Heart Protector allows us to be open-hearted and loving without being overly sensitive to emotional hurts.

The "Three Heater" is responsible for regulating our temperature. It makes sure that we are not too hot or too cold and that each part of our body is warm enough. Like the Heart Protector, it does not have a specific organ associated with it. It governs perspiration as well as our ability to generate sufficient heat to keep us warm. It also provides us with the warmth and balance we need to interact effectively with our family, friends, and the rest of the world.

Earth Element

Late Summer

The official in charge of digestion, the Stomach official, takes in nourishment from our Mother Earth and breaks it down into its simple, essential components so that we can absorb what is useful. It gives us the ability to take in information as well and the ability to feel and appreciate the abundance of life.

Our Spleen official is responsible for the distribution of nourishment and chi throughout our whole system. It moves our mind and spirit as well so we do not get stuck ruminating and obsessing.

Metal Element

Autumn

The Lung official, or "Receiver of the Heavenly Chi," absorbs energy from the air we breathe. It also provides clarity, inspiration, and quality of life from our Heavenly Father.

The "Drainer of the Dregs," our Colon official, eliminates the physical as well as mental and spiritual garbage from the day before, including confusion, misconceptions, grudges, hatreds, regrets, prejudices, and so on.

Law of Midday/Midnight

Another aspect of the daily ebb and flow of chi throughout our system is the Law of Midday/Midnight. Each of the internal organs receives more energy during one two-hour period of the day and decidedly less twelve hours later. It is like a tide of energy moving through our system.

In addition to the time of day when each official receives more energy, each receives more energy during the time of year that corresponds to its element.

The Chinese Clock chart below show each of the twelve officials with its most energetic time of day, most active time of year, corresponding element, and primary function.

The Chinese Clock

Official	Peak Time	Season	Element	Primary Function
Lungs	3–5 a.m.	Autumn	Metal	Receiving the Heavenly Chi
Colon	5–7 a.m.	Autumn	Metal	Draining the Dregs
Stomach	7–9 a.m.	Late Summer	Earth	Digestion
Spleen	9–11 a.m.	Late Summer	Earth	Transportation
Heart	11 a.m.–1 p.m.	Summer	Fire	Supreme Controller
Small Intestine	1–3 p.m.	Summer	Fire	Sorting Pure from Impure
Bladder	3–5 p.m.	Winter	Water	Properly Storing Fluids
Kidneys	5–7 p.m.	Winter	Water	Purifying and Distributing Fluids
Heart Protector	7–9 p.m.	Summer	Fire	Circulation and Sexual Energy
Three Heater	9–11 p.m.	Summer	Fire	Even Distribution of Warmth
Gall Bladder	11p.m.–1 a.m.	Spring	Wood	Decision Making
Liver	1–3 a.m.	Spring	Wood	Planning

All times of day listed in the Chinese Clock chart are sun time, not daylight savings time. Each element has two officials except the Fire Element, which has four.

Understanding the officials and when they are naturally at their peak of efficiency is useful for two reasons. First, it can help us understand why we may have a time of day when we feel our best and a time when we feel we are dragging. The variation in our energy level over the course of the day can be an indication of which of the officials is getting too much or too little energy. For example, if your chi is backed up in your Decision Maker and Great Planner, you may find it hard to fall asleep (or to stay asleep) when they get even more energy between 11 p.m. and 3 a.m.

Second, understanding the Chinese Clock can help us live more in harmony with the natural cycles that occur within us. We can use it to help us balance our chi and help us use our energy efficiently.

Early in the morning, when your Receiver of the Heavenly Chi is at its peak and when the air is fresh and clean, get out for a walk or do your breathing meditations. Take in an abundant wave of energy from the air, sometimes referred to as the "lead chi," to carry you through the day.

Allow time for a leisurely visit to the bathroom between 5 and 7 a.m., and many bowel problems will improve. So will your ability to let go of whatever disappointments and frustrations you felt the day before so you can start the day with a clean slate.

Have your main meal, or at least a substantial, nourishing breakfast, between 7 and 9 a.m. It will provide the fuel to carry you through the day. Unfortunately, many people have their main meal in the evening, when their stomach is trying to rest. No wonder their bowels are likely to be off and they have little appetite in the morning, when their stomach is still dealing with stale food from the night before. Eat a light dinner, and you will likely lose weight and feel better in the morning.

Eat well for breakfast, and you will have much better energy throughout the day.

Make sure you get plenty of water to drink, especially if you feel a dip in your energy level in the afternoon. Remember the general guideline of dividing your weight (in pounds) in half and drinking that many fluid ounces of water (not including coffee, tea, or juice) each day. Have a light supper. If your sexual energy is not what you would like it to be, rather than a big evening meal, take advantage of your sexual energy's high point between 7 and 9 p.m.

If you want some alcohol in the evening, allow time for your system to metabolize it before you head off to bed. The Decision Maker and Great Planner function best without any external input, as their work is internal. Sleep on your right side, so they are bathed in blood while they are most active. When facing an important decision, follow the old adage, "Let me sleep on it." Allow these officials to provide much wiser plans and decisions than your thinking mind will produce.

I encourage you to adjust your routines to take advantage of the times of day when each official is functioning at its peak and the times when each is, relatively speaking, at rest. Put this information to the test for a month and see how you feel.

Chapter 13

Following the Tao

Following the Tao involves understanding and living in harmony with the natural laws that govern how the creation functions. Fundamental to this is developing an awareness of our essential, timeless nature. This is a big task. Because our level of awareness determines everything we do, I have come to see abiding in an awareness of our true nature as a main goal of life.

There are many different paths to following the Tao and cultivating our chi, some more suited to one person than another. Regardless, there are principles common to them and stages along the path:

1. blindly believing one's unexamined assumptions and routinely anesthetizing oneself using favorite chi burners to ease the pain they produce;

2. realizing one's unexamined assumptions are the cause of one's suffering; and

3. experiencing and then stabilizing an ongoing awareness of one's essential self.

Life has its ups and downs regardless of one's level of awareness, but my experience is that the more aware I am the less buffeted about and the more relaxed I feel.

The stages along the way are fixed and predictable. They apply to all of us. Understanding these stages and being able to see where we are along the way is an enormous help in self-observation. The first stage of starting to wake up is disillusionment. This is a precarious stage because it can be so painful. One can easily turn to drugs, alcohol, or suicide.

Seeing someone go through this is unsettling. It is tempting to try to cheer the person up and help him or her return to normal. Family and friends, distressed at seeing a loved one feel acutely unhappy, often exert considerable pressure to seek medications. We tend to feel more comfortable when everyone seems happy, believing the same cultural norms and beliefs, regardless of how dysfunctional those beliefs may be and how much suffering they may cause.

There is little understanding in our culture for the disillusionment that precedes beginning a serious effort to become more balanced and more aware. Disillusionment is the necessary prerequisite to realizing that our lack of awareness of our essential nature is the cause of our suffering. It is an opportunity to begin a serious path towards waking up and regaining our balance. Rather than try to escape it, I encourage you to use it to move towards greater balance and awareness of your real needs.

Next comes an interest in understanding the natural laws about consciousness. Several paths work with knowledge about these laws. Arica offers one, Buddhism provides another. T'ai Chi, Sufism, and Taoism are among additional possibilities. The knowledge they convey is based on observation and experience.

Applying these principles of consciousness has opened the way for me to understand and more easily repeat experiencing the interconnectedness of all the creation. Singing or playing music together can produce the feeling of being at one with others. Feeling the warm breeze and the sun while listening to the waves on the beach can calm one's thinking mind sufficiently to allow for feeling at one with nature. Playing on a sports team, where the teamwork is really happening, can produce it. Psychotropic drugs can temporarily produce it. So can sex, dancing, or zipping down a mountain on your skis when you are perfectly in the flow.

This feeling of being at one comes and goes. Although many activities can produce a flash of it, having it become our normal state is another matter. The main difficulty is the rude and unexpected intrusion of thoughts or feelings that our mind insists are real and that urgently need our attention. It can be an abrupt transition from being relaxed and in the flow to feeling angry, sad, or fearful, all because something triggered an unpleasant thought or feeling.

An effective path toward being awake must have a means of examining the thoughts that arise, seeing their root, and seeing them as our mind's interpretation of the sensory information we have noticed. It will, sooner or later, necessitate reviewing our past experiences, from which we have formed our basic assumptions and beliefs about life.

Reviewing our past can stir up a lot of emotions. An effective means of making peace with our past experiences and appreciating what we have learned as a result is necessary. Otherwise, examining emotionally charged experiences from our past can be a lot like picking a scab, opening the wound again and prolonging the time needed to heal.

I've come to see that learning from our past experiences has several components. We learn what works and what doesn't as we become more capable and proficient. We learn what suits us and what doesn't. We learn how to avoid unpleasant experiences and repeat pleasant ones.

The most transformative learning is finding that no matter our circumstances, our essential self remains unchanged. It simply observes our experience.

Seeing our experiences and our reactions to them from this vantage deepens our ability to see the unborn, timeless, and eternal presence of the Divine in ourselves and everyone else. It is the foundation of real compassion. This awareness gives us the ability to let go of the emotional charge and resulting tensions and out-of-balance desires we carry from our past experiences.

The Arica *Nine Hypergnostic Systems*™ training provides a complete and efficient means of reviewing our past experiences and meditations to make peace with them and use them to help awaken our awareness of the presence of the Divine in each of us.

I have found the main difficulty in daily cultivating my chi and following the Tao according to the seasons and time of day is my compulsion to try to accomplish something, to fill an imaginary need or shortcoming from my past, or to avoid repeating unpleasant or threatening experiences I have had.

The odd and dysfunctional thing about indulging this compulsion is that it can result in neglecting my T'ai Chi or meditation practice. I want to start work earlier or end work later than I should. Sometimes, whatever I want to accomplish seems more important than my daily practice. Getting sick can be a reminder that cultivating my chi is as important a part of my daily routine as eating, sleeping, and brushing my teeth.

Chasing my ambitions and ignoring my most essential needs is such a contradiction that any sane person would have a good laugh over it.

Sometimes, I do.

Common Knowledge, Common Sense

If I had read this book when I was eighteen—young, strong, healthy, a politically conservative member of the church, playing music in a hot soul band, and racing my motorcycle—I would have thought the author was crazy. Many of the ideas presented here would have been so foreign to me and so different from what I believed to be true that I would have rejected them outright. While I could see contradictions in my beliefs,

I harbored no doubt that the common knowledge upon which my worldview was based was essentially accurate.

When I was twenty-one, so many aspects of my life seemed to fail simultaneously and I felt so upset by these events that I began to question my fundamental assumptions about life. I was fortunate to find a path for examining my core beliefs and assumptions and recognizing that many of them were not absolute truth, but simply a construction of my mind. I was blessed that my family and friends, while at times wondering what I was doing, were nonetheless supportive.

I was most fortunate to encounter and learn from the extraordinary teachers who shared, for the benefit of all people, the concepts and practices mentioned in this book. My experience over the past thirty-seven years has, time and again, confirmed what I have learned from them.

Some of what is in this book may be a new way of seeing things for you, as most of it was for me. Although spiritual in the sense of recognizing that all is a manifestation of the One, this book is about awareness, not religion. The wisdom shared in this book is simply about the immutable natural laws governing the creation and how to live in harmony with each other and the world around us. These ideas have deepened my understanding and appreciation of the heart of every religion I have encountered that teaches love, compassion, and the Golden Rule.

Doing our best to understand and follow the fundamental laws of nature now seems like common sense to me. We feel best with fresh food that grows nearby and in season. We need enough water each day. Breathing slowly and deeply gives us more energy and helps us relax. Relaxing and living in harmony with the seasons and the times of day helps us use our energy more efficiently.

Fundamental to relaxing is remembering our timeless nature and easing our death grip on basic assumptions that are unrealistic and make us feel alone, at odds with those around us, and separate from nature. While medications can be lifesaving, staying on them when we could change how we live, regain our health, and let go of those medications hastens our decline. A daily practice, based on the natural laws that govern how to nourish our chi, is enjoyable and indispensable to feeling our best.

Time of Change

We live in a time of unprecedented change. Advances in science and manufacturing, coupled with decades of cheap oil, gave us the ability to rapidly reshape the world before fully understanding the consequences. The resulting climate change, depletion of our soil, industrialization of our food sources, tampering with nature's genetic blueprint, extinction of other species that play a vital part in the balance of life, and pollution of our water and air are producing a great increase in severe diseases affecting our bodies, mental clarity, and will to live.

We can now measure and track the changes we have set in motion, and we can communicate what we see instantly throughout the world. As we awaken to the reality of our situation and the dangers to our survival we now face, we can see that unbridled self-interest and corporate greed are no longer viable options. Recognizing and letting go of an old ethic that encourages them and of the fears and unexamined beliefs at the root of this ethic are difficult tasks.

Ignorance of the interconnectedness of all life is not a viable option anymore either, nor is pretending we are not aware of the consequences of what we are doing. We must do our best to understand and live in harmony with nature, including our bodies and those around us.

We must be willing to see and respond to our situation as it is in its totality.

As Chief Seattle reputedly said in 1854:

> This we know. The earth does not belong to man; man belongs to the earth. Whatever befalls the earth befalls the sons of the earth. This we know. All things are connected like the blood that unites one family. All things are connected.[1]

Twenty-five hundred years ago, Confucius, in *The Great Learning,* wrote that when the ancients wanted to restore balance and harmony to the world, they first had to restore balance and harmony to their state. Before they could restore balance and harmony to their state, it was necessary to restore balance and harmony to their province, and before that to their city. Before that could be accomplished, they needed to bring balance and harmony to their neighborhood, and before that to their family. One could not hope to bring balance and harmony to their family without first gaining mastery over their own life. So, the way to restore balance and harmony to the world begins with restoring balance and harmony to one's own self.

I hope this book helps you in cultivating a way of life that is balanced, realistic, joyful, and healthy.

Chapter Notes

[1] Shelley Tucker, *Openings: Quotations on Spirituality in Everyday Life,* 49. While there are varying opinions on how accurately Chief Seattle's comments were recorded and translated, the truth of this statement is undeniable.

Hall of Happiness

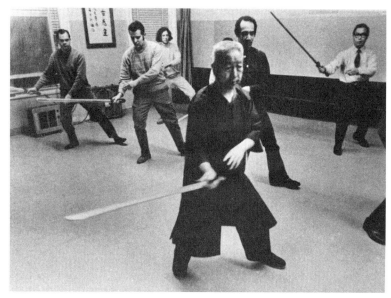

Professor Cheng Man-Ch'ing. (Photo courtesy of Kenneth Van Sickle.)

T he following inscription hangs over the door to Prof Cheng's Shr Jung T'ai Chi School in New York City.

May the joy that is everlasting gather in this hall.

Not the joy of a sumptuous feast, which slips quickly away even as we leave the table, nor that which music brings—it is only of limited duration.

Beauty and a pretty face are like flowers; they bloom for a while then die. Even our youth slips swiftly away and is gone. No, enduring happiness is not in these nor the Three Joys of Jung Kung. We may as well forget them, for the joy I am speaking of is worlds away from these.

It is the joy of continuous growth, of helping to develop in ourselves and others the talents and abilities with which we were born—the gifts of heaven to mortal men. It is to revive the exhausted and rejuvenate that which is in decline, so that we are able to dispel sickness and suffering.

Let true affection and happy concourse abide in this Hall.

Let us here correct our past mistakes and lose our preoccupation with self. With the constancy of the planets in their courses and the dragon in its cloud-wrapped path, let us enter the land of health and ever after walk within its bounds. Let us fortify ourselves against weakness and learn to be self-reliant without a moment's lapse. Then our resolution will become the very air we breathe, the world we live in; then we will be as happy as fish in crystal waters.

This is the joy that lasts, that we can carry with us to the end of our days. And tell me, if you can, what greater joy can life bestow.

Appendix

If we are serious about nourishing our chi, some fundamental awareness and knowledge of what we are eating and how it got to our table is essential. Michael Pollan's book, *The Omnivore's Dilemma,* is a great help, as is the film, *Food, Inc.*, directed by Robert Kenner.

The following pages outline some additional information about food that is worth considering when cultivating a more healthy life.

Eat Your Vegetables

The relatively low cost of meat and dairy products, made possible by industrialized farming, has shifted what we eat heavily in the direction of animal protein sources, much more than we need and far more than is healthy for us. T. Colin Campbell, PhD, in his book, *The China Study*, shares the conclusions of the China-Oxford-Cornell Diet and Health Project, a twenty-year study done by Cornell University, the University of Oxford, and the Chinese Academy of Preventive Medicine. Called the "Grand Prix of epidemiology" and the "most comprehensive large study ever undertaken of the relationship between diet and the risk of developing disease" by the *New York Times*, his book details the connections between nutrition and diabetes, heart disease, and cancer. This study showed incidence of the above diseases up to twenty times higher among those who ate the most meat and dairy products compared to those whose diet was predominately plant based.

Sugars

Plants use energy from the sun to make two simple sugars—glucose and fructose. We extract these two simple sugars to make refined white sugar, high fructose corn syrup, and other high fructose sweeteners. White sugar is 50 percent glucose and 50 percent fructose. High fructose sweeteners simply contain more fructose than glucose.

According to the July 2012 USDA report, "Sugar and Sweetener Outlook,"[1] the average per capita consumption of refined sugar, high fructose corn syrup, and other high fructose sweeteners in the United States during 2011 exceeded 130 pounds. This includes, in addition to the refined white sugar we put in our coffee, shockingly high amounts of sugar and high fructose sweeteners in baby formula as well as in sodas, juices, soft drinks, sports drinks, baby food, candy, ice cream, pastries, yogurt, peanut butter, cookies, bread, ketchup, mustard and other condiments, sauces, salad dressings, crackers, chips, and countless other prepared foods.

Health problems that are much more severe than previously understood arise from consuming refined sugar, high fructose corn syrup, and other high fructose sweeteners. In May of 2009, Robert Lustig, MD, UCSF Professor of Pediatrics in the Division of Endocrinology, gave a lecture, titled "Sugar: The Bitter Truth," which was posted on the UCSF education website on May 26, 2009. It describes what happens inside us when we consume refined sugar, high fructose corn syrup, and high fructose sweeteners. A web link to the lecture is listed in the Resources section at the end of this book.

To summarize the effects of sugar on our body, while every cell in our body metabolizes glucose, fructose is primarily metabolized in the liver. When the liver receives a big jolt of fructose from baby formula, fruit juice, a soft drink, candy, a sugary pastry, honey, agave, maple syrup, and so on, it maintains equilibrium in our system by quickly converting the fructose to fat, in particular, the Pattern B LDL (small molecule "bad" cholesterol) that sticks tenaciously to arterial walls and forms plaque.

The production and accumulation of this type of fat also leads to a metabolic disorder where our cells lose the ability to respond to normal insulin levels. Simultaneously, fructose impedes the feedback loop that tells us when we have sufficient glucose in our blood and it's time to stop eating. Still feeling hungry, we continue eating more than we need.

The excess food further heightens our blood sugar level. Our pancreas must produce more insulin to control it. The presence of high levels of fructose creates a vicious cycle of overeating and increasing cellular resistance to insulin, resulting in the need for more and more insulin to control the blood sugar level. When your pancreas can no longer keep up, you get Type II diabetes and/or another condition known as "metabolic syndrome," characterized by weight gain, particularly around the belly, heightened levels of Pattern B LDL, arterial plaque, and high blood pressure.

High insulin levels and the attendant high levels of insulin growth factor (IGF) are also a potent trigger for healthy cells becoming cancerous and a powerful accelerant for cancer growth. David Servan-Schreiber, MD, PhD, wrote in his book, *Anti-Cancer: A New Way of Life,* that researchers at Harvard and UCSF have noted increases of up to 700 percent in the incidence of breast cancer and 900 percent for prostate cancer in patients with the highest IGF levels. Even high-starch/low-fiber content products made with refined flour can cause spikes in blood sugar levels sufficient to significantly increase the risk of many cancers.

Finally, although I am not aware of any research or statistics on the relationship of sugar to arthritis, several patients and students who have suffered from severe arthritis have reported that when they don't consume refined sugar and high fructose sweeteners they have much less pain, stiffness, and inflammation.

Putting aside foods and drinks laden with refined sugar and high fructose sweeteners in favor of abundant fruit, vegetables, legumes, and whole grains is a great help in avoiding and recovering from the diseases caused by toxic sweeteners.

Genetically Modified Foods

When I first heard there are serious questions about the safety of genetically modified (GM) crops, also known as genetically modified organisms (GMOs), I was skeptical, reasoning that humans have been cross-pollinating and grafting plants for thousands of years, to our great benefit. Over time, seeing an increasing number of patients with severe allergies, illness related to their immune systems, as well as digestive and other disorders, I began to pay more attention.

I found that GMOs are not produced by the benign traditional means of grafting and cross-pollination or by the safe, modern, and effective means of Marker Assisted Selection that facilitates specific trait selection from within the same species. These traditional methods of refining a crop's usefulness rely on the exchange of genetic material within various strains of the same species of plant. Genes from a corn plant that has a desirable trait, for example, replace genes from another strain of corn that lacks the desired trait.

Genetic modification employs a completely different method to force bits of genetic code from bacteria, viruses, and other life forms that are foreign to the crop's species into its genome. As of this writing, there are four basic steps:

1. Select and isolate the genes that will produce the desired trait, either from a virus, bacteria, plant, animal, or artificial source.

2. Add additional bacterial or viral code to the ends of the selected genes (these bacterial or viral genes are necessary to activate the inserted genes).

3. Fracture the host's genetic sequence and force the newly created gene sequence into the host's genome, permanently altering its genetic code.

4. Test to see whether the host is still viable and, if so, exhibits the desired trait.

Testing for safety is not among these steps. According to *GMO Myths and Truths*,[2] written in June 2012 by Michael Antoniou, Claire Robinson, and John Fagan, genetic modification is dangerous for a number of reasons summarized below.

Firstly, our immune systems have evolved over thousands of years to recognize viruses, bacteria, and other life forms that don't belong in our bodies as foreign invaders that threaten our life. A healthy immune system, confronted with such an invader, mounts an immune response designed to eliminate the invader. This may include coughing, runny nose, diarrhea, fever, swelling, vomiting, and producing antibodies that trigger a systemic immune response, clumping the invaders together, triggering production of immune cells, and summoning these cells to gobble up the invader.

Bits of genetic code from the bacteria, viruses, or other sources of new code forced into the host cell's genome cause the host to produce proteins and polysaccharides known as antigens, which have characteristics of the donor virus, bacteria, or other species. Some people's bodies are more selective than others about what they accept and what their immune system sees as a foreign invader. Antigens can cause allergic reactions if our immune system recognizes them as alien and potentially harmful. When an antigen accompanies genetically modified corn, wheat, soy, or an otherwise safe and healthy food were it not for the GMO components within it, a person's immune response may develop antibodies that trigger a reaction to future exposures to that food even if it is non-GMO. In other words, if your immune system is triggered by eating genetically modified corn, wheat, or soy, you can become allergic to non-GMO corn, wheat, and soy as well.

A growing body of evidence strongly suggests that GMO crops and the associated herbicides they require are contributing to the increase of immune system illnesses, including food and other allergies, as well as other disorders, especially among children. Even for those who are healthy now, I believe there are strong risks with chronically challenging one's immune system with GMO antigens and accompanying chemical residues.

Secondly, while cross-pollination, grafting, and Marker Assisted Selection do not disrupt the sequence of genetic material in a crop's genome, genetic modification does. It is not yet possible to fracture a host cell's DNA and then insert genes for a desired trait into a specific place on its genetic sequence. Where the inserted gene ends up in the DNA chain of the host cell's genome (i.e., where in relation to its neighboring genes) is random. This is significant because the various genes in an organism's genome do not act in a linear way, with each gene producing only one specific protein. They work in combinations. Changing one gene is likely to produce, in addition to the desired trait, a number of unintended additional traits as the newly inserted genetically modified genes interact with their neighbors instead of the genes that would normally occupy that position on the host cell's genome. The resulting proteins the cell produces can be toxic, allergenic, destructive, or unable to perform an essential function. Simply disrupting the sequence in which bits of genetic code appear, even without adding foreign code, alters their function in a number of unpredictable ways that can be harmful and may not be apparent until much later.

Mounting evidence suggests proteins produced by GMOs do interfere with normal development and/or disrupt normal functions, especially in fetal and early childhood development. Unlike food poisoning, which becomes obvious and traceable within a short time, these developmental disruptions can be severe, remain hidden for years, and permanently affect the developing child and his or her offspring.

The interactions of the genetic components of a cell's genome are interrelated and very complex. Consequently, changes from even one genetic modification trigger additional changes that are almost impossible to predict or track, even with careful research. Releasing genetically modified plants into the environment where their pollen will spread and they will be eaten by other species has consequences, whether beneficial or harmful, that may not be known for years.

Finally, some of the toxins genetically modified crops are bred to produce to ward off insects can cause severe digestive inflammation. Since these toxins are inside the genetically modified cells, they cannot be washed off.

When genetically modified crops first appeared, the FDA, against the advice of its own scientists, yielded to corporate pressure in deciding to entrust all testing for the safety of genetically modified crops to the corporations that produce them. The FDA still does not test genetically modified crops for safety. European safety standards are only slightly stronger. No credible long-term testing for genetically modified crop safety has been done. Fearing an informed public might not accept genetically modified foods when they were first introduced,

GMO producers also prevailed in preventing government requirements to list genetically modified ingredients, making it difficult for consumers to choose or avoid them, and for researchers to track their safety.

Rhetoric aside, the actions of the corporations that produce genetically modified crops and the herbicides and pesticides these crops require has made it clear that maximizing sales is their primary concern. Consumer safety is not. In fact, numerous independent studies have shown significantly more tumors, developmental and neurological problems, and diseases affecting the liver, kidneys, gonads, stomach, intestines, and other internal organs of laboratory animals raised on genetically modified crops compared to those raised on non-GMOs. Similar effects on food-producing animals are known and are suspected on humans.

While genetically modified crops may someday fulfill the promise of safe, hardier, higher yield, more nutritious, more pest-resistant strains that require less herbicide and pesticide use compared with more traditional varieties, to date these have not proven true. Associated herbicide and pesticide use is increasing as weeds and insects are becoming resistant to the new strains and accompanying chemicals.

Meanwhile, we continue to be unwitting subjects of a vast, uncontrolled experiment with potentially dangerous consequences. Rigorous, long-term, third-party testing for public and environmental safety is needed before approving genetically modified crops for distribution. Open sharing of information, starting with labeling genetically modified crops and foods with GMO ingredients so that consumers can make informed choices, should also be a requirement. If GMOs really are better, instead of spending 44 million dollars in a successful bid to defeat California's recent Proposition 37 initiative to require labeling of GMO containing foods, those who produce them ought to be proud to label GMO foods so consumers can more easily find and buy them.

Until then, Terry Cook's advice on avoiding GMOs is well founded. Unless a food is labeled "non-GM", "non-GMO" or "Organic", chances are it contains ingredients from genetically modified crops and there is no way for consumers to tell.

Hormone-mimicking Toxins

Some of the wraps and packaging around our food are also toxic. For example, PVC is a type of plastic commonly used in food packaging, plastic baby bottles and sippy cups, some types of soft-drink bottles, cups, utensils, and the white plastic linings of cans. When it comes in contact with hot foods, these plastic containers release biphenyl A, a toxic, carcinogenic, estrogen-mimicking organic chemical in the PVC, which diffuses into the food.

A recent experiment at Harvard found that eating a single serving per day for one week of a popular brand of vegetable soup, packaged in cans lined with PVC, resulted in blood levels of biphenyl A one thousand times higher than a control group eating the same soup for one week from cans not lined with PVC.

Biphenyl A is particularly toxic to fetuses and infants, where it can disrupt neurological development and contribute to autism, which has become far more common among children than it was a generation ago.

Summary

Although there are dietary recommendations for specific health concerns, and many dietary fads have come and gone, the simple truth remains that our bodies are highly evolved to use the food that nature provides for us. Our recent attempts at genetic modification to improve these foods and industrializing their production degrade their quality and are often dangerous. Old fashioned, locally grown, organic whole foods are a much safer, more reliable source of vitality and nutrition. It's a good bet they taste better, too.

Chapter Notes

1   http://www.ers.usda.gov/publications/sssm-sugar-and-sweeteners-outlook/sssm273.aspx

2 http://www.earthopensource.org/files/pdfs/GMO Myths and Truths/GMO Myths and Truths 1.3a.pdf

Resources

For further information you may contact:

- Arica Institute (www.arica.org) for a complete description of the Arica School and available trainings.

- The Five Element Acupuncture Community website (www.feacom.com) for a complete listing of schools and practitioners of Classical Five Element Acupuncture.

- Long River T'ai Chi Circle (www.longrivertaichi.org/cmclineagelist.htm) for a listing of teachers and schools teaching T'ai Chi as taught by Cheng Man-ch'ing.

- The T'ai Chi Foundation (www.taichifoundation.org) for a complete listing of schools using the teaching method developed by Patrick Watson to teach T'ai Chi Chuan as he learned it from Cheng Man-ch'ing and the recently completed *Roots and Branches Five Element Qi Gong* DVD.

- Institute for Functional Medicine (www.functional-medicine.org), and the American Dietetic Association (www.eatright.org) for listings of qualified dieticians and nutritionists.

I suggest the following books, articles, DVDs, and lecture:

Antoniou, Michael, Claire Robinson, and John Fagan. *GMO Myths and Truths*. Earth Open Source.org, 2012

Brandt, Edna, and Pat Gorman, *How to Cultivate Your Chi*. New York: T'ai Chi Press Magazine, Volume II No. IV, the School of T'ai Chi Chuan, 1990.

Brody, Jane E. "A Downside to T'ai Chi? None That I See." Health Section, *New York Times*, September 28, 2010.

Campbell, T. Colin, PhD. *The China Study*, Jackson, Tennessee: The China Study and BenBella Books, Inc., 2009.

Cheng Man Ch'ing. *Cheng Tzu's Thirteen Treatises on T'ai Chi Ch'uan*. Translated by Benjamin Pang Jeng Lo and Martin Inn. Berkeley, California: North Atlantic Books, 1985.

Cheng Man-jan. *Lao-Tzu: "My words are very easy to understand."* Lectures on the Tao Teh Ching. Translated by Tam C. Gibbs. Richmond, California: North Atlantic Books, 1981.

Goodell, David. *Cultivating Your Chi*, DVD. Seattle, Washington: Center for Classical Five Element Acupuncture, 2009.

Gorman, Pat, *Roots and Branches Five Element Qi Gong*, DVD. New York: T'ai Chi Foundation, 2011.

Ichazo, Oscar. *The Human Process for Enlightenment and Freedom*. New York: Arica Institute, 1975.

———. *Master Level Exercise: Psychocalisthenics*. New York: Sequoia Press, 1986.

Kenner, Robert and Eric Schlosser. *Food, Inc., DVD*. New York: Magnolia Pictures, 2008. http://www.foodinc-movie.com/

Lustig, Robert, MD. "Sugar: The Bitter Truth." Lecture given on July 27, 2009 at UC San Francisco. (www.uctv.tv/search-details.aspx?showID=16717)

Lowenthal, Wolfe. *Gateway to the Miraculous: Further Explorations in the Tao of Cheng Man-ch'ing*. Berkeley, California: Frog, Ltd.,1994.

———. *Like a Long River: Some T'ai Chi Thoughts*. Amherst, Massachusetts: Long River T'ai Chi Press, 2005.

———. *There Are No Secrets: Professor Cheng Man-ch'ing and his T'ai Chi Chuan*, Berkeley, California: Frog, Ltd., 1991.

Pollan, Michael. *The Omnivore's Dilemma: A Natural History of Four Meals*. New York: Penguin Press, 2006.

Servan-Schreiber, David, MD, PhD. *Anti Cancer—A New Way of Life*. New York: Viking Penguin, 2009.

Tucker, Shelly. *Openings: Quotations on Spirituality in Everyday Life*. Seattle, Washington: Whiteaker Press, 1997.

Worsley, J. R. *Talking about Acupuncture in New York*. Church Hill Farm, England: Worsley Inc., 2004.

Acknowledgements

I want to acknowledge and thank:

Oscar Ichazo, originator of the Arica Theory and Method for the Attainment of Pristine Enlightenment and founder of Arica Institute, and Sarah Ichazo for their teaching, inspiration, and feedback.

Professor Cheng Man-ch'ing, founder of Shr Jung T'ai Chi School.

Patrick Watson, founder of the School of T'ai Chi Chuan and the T'ai Chi Foundation.

J. R. Worsley and Judy Becker Worsley, my principle acupuncture teachers.

Also:

Roy Capellaro, RPT, Zero Balancing teacher and practitioner, for his wisdom and advice.

Terry Cook, PhD, for her contribution to this book about genetic modification and her advice and review of the information about GMOs presented in the Appendix.

Lori Annaheim, Gene Giffen, Rita Goodell, Pat Gorman, Patti Hulvershorn, Carolyn Mueller, Samantha Nolloth, and Charles Thompson, MD, for their editing assistance.

Pat Gorman, MAc, for her advice and encouragement.

April Hulvershorn, MAc, for her inspiration, encouragement, editing assistance and advice.

Eliot Ivanhoe, MD, MAc, for the talk he gave presenting a continuum of health.

Margaret Matsumoto, director of Teacher Training for the T'ai Chi Foundation, for her wisdom, editing assistance, and advice.

John Shackford for editing.

My family and friends for their generosity and open-mindedness.

About the Author

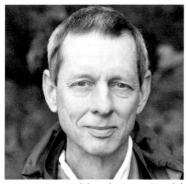

(Photo by Poppy Barach.)

The eldest of five sons of John and Esther Goodell, David was born in Jamestown, New York, in 1951. He especially enjoyed swimming, boating, skiing, other outdoor sports, and playing music. He earned his living as a bassist in various working bands in western New York until moving to Arlington, Virginia, in 1975 to participate in Arica work there. By 1976, he was also studying T'ai Chi with The School of T'ai Chi Chuan, Inc., founded by Patrick Watson.

While completing the necessary pre-med courses to study acupuncture, he also earned a bachelor's degree in Chinese Civilization from George Mason University in 1983. He graduated from the Traditional Acupuncture Institute (TAI) in Columbia, Maryland, in 1985 and has maintained a private practice in Classical Five Element Acupuncture since.

Recognizing that proficiency comes from experience accompanied by ongoing study, he continued his acupuncture studies with J. R. Worsley, earning his BAc (UK) from the College of Traditional Acupuncture, UK, in 1989; MAc from the TAI in 1990; and AcM (UK) in 1996. He organized and attended numerous Patient Consultation Days and Seminars with J. R. and Judy Worsley. David is a graduate and was a coaching assistant in their Basic and Advanced Teacher Training programs. He was a clinical supervisor at TAI from 1995–1997. He was a participant in the Worsley's Master Apprentice Program from its inception in 1997 until 2008, serving as a senior coach from 2002–2008. He was a founding member and president of the Worsley Institute, a non-profit educational organization, from 1998–2008.

Meanwhile, David continued to study and teach T'ai Chi with the School of T'ai Chi Chuan and continued his meditation and acupuncture practice. Within a year of moving to Seattle in 2005, he established the Seattle School of T'ai Chi (www.taichiseattle.com) and, shortly after, co-founded the Center for Classical Five Element Acupuncture (www.centercfea.com) with his wife, April Hulvershorn. April and David both practice acupuncture at the Center for Classical Five Element Acupuncture.

In cooperation with colleagues Eliot Ivanhoe, MD, MAc, and Neil Gumenick, MAc, David helps plan the annual Five Element Acupuncture Symposiums, organized and hosted by Neil's school, the Institute of Five Element Acupuncture.

He recently established the Five Element Acupuncture Community website (www.feacom.com) as a service to the public and to the acupuncture community. This site hosts a comprehensive practitioner referral list and numerous videotaped presentations from the Five-Element Acupuncture Symposiums and related events. DVDs on aspects of T'ai Chi and related healing arts are also available on this site.

This book is available directly from the
Center for Classical Five Element Acupuncture
www.centercfea.com
206-298-9376.